BUILDING REGIONAL HEALTH CARE NETWORKS IN EUROPE

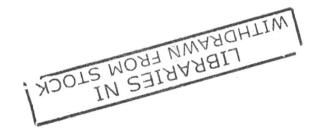

Studies in Health Technology and Informatics

Editors

Jens Pihlkjaer Christensen, European Commission DG XIII/C-5, Brussels; Tim De Dombal †, University of Leeds;
Ilias Iakovidis, EC DG XIII Health Telematics, Brussels; Zoi Kolitsi, University of Patras;
Jaap Noothoven van Goor †, ACOSTA, Brussels; Antonio Pedotti, Politecnico di·Milan; Otto Rienhoff,
Georg-August-Universität Göttingen; Francis H. Roger France, Centre for Medical Informatics, UCL, Brussels;
Niels Rossing, Centre for Clinical Imaging and Engineering, National University Hospital, Copenhagen;
Faina Shtern, National Institutes of Health, Bethesda, MD; Viviane Thévenin, CEC DG XII/F BIOMED-I,
Brussels

Volume 67

Earlier published in this series

Vol. 35. M. Di Rienzo, G. Mancia, G. Parati, A. Pedotti and A. Zanchetti (Eds.), Frontiers of Blood Pressure and Heart Rate Analysis

Vol. 36. M. Sosa-ludicissa, N. Oliveri, C.A. Gamboa and J. Roberts (Eds.), Internet, Telematics and Health

Vol. 37. J.A. Sevastik and K.M. Diab (Eds.), Research into Spinal Deformities 1

Vol. 38. R.A. Mortensen (Ed.), ICNP in Europe: TELENURSE

Vol. 39. K.S. Morgan, H.M. Hoffman, D. Stredney and S.J. Weghorst (Eds.), Medicine Meets Virtual Reality

Vol. 40. G. Lowet, P. Rüegsegger, H. Weinans and A. Meunier (Eds.), Bone Research in Biomechanics

Vol. 41. J. Mantas (Ed.), Health Telematics Education

Vol. 42. J. Brender, Methodology for Assessment of Medical IT-Based Systems

Vol. 43. C. Pappas, N. Maglaveras and J.-R. Scherrer (Eds.), Medical Informatics Europe '97

Vol. 44. G. Riva (Ed.), Virtual Reality in Neuro-Psycho-Physiology

Vol. 45. J. Dudeck, B. Blobel, W. Lordieck and T. Bürkle (Eds.), New Technologies in Hospital Information Systems

Vol. 46. U. Gerdin, M. Tallberg and P. Wainwright (Eds.), Nursing Informatics

Vol. 47. W. Ceusters, P. Spyns, G. De Moor and W. Martin (Eds.), Syntactic-Semantic Tagging of Medical Texts: The Multi-TALE Project

Vol. 48. J. Graafmans, V. Taipale and N. Charness (Eds.), Gerontechnology

Vol. 49. L. van den Broek and A.J. Sikkel (Eds.), Health Cards '97

Vol. 50. J.D. Westwood, H.M. Hoffman, D. Stredney and S.J. Weghorst (Eds.), Medicine Meets Virtual Reality

Vol. 51. J. Mantas (Ed.), Advances in Health Telematics Education

Vol. 52. B. Cesnik, A.T. McCray and J.-R. Scherrer (Eds.), MedInfo '98

Vol. 53. M.C. Sievert, D.E. Moxley, N.J. Ogg and T.B. Patrick, Thesaurus of Health Informatics

Vol. 54. O. Ferrer-Roca and M. Sosa-Iudicissa (Eds.), Handbook of Telemedicine

Vol. 55. H.M.J. Goldschmidt, M.J.T. Cox, R.J.E. Grouls, W.A.J.H. van de Laar and G.G. van Merode, Reference Information Model for Clinical Laboratories

Vol. 56. I. Iakovidis, S. Maglavera and A. Trakatellis (Eds.), User Acceptance of Health Telematics Applications

Vol. 57. J. Mantas (Ed.), Health and Medical Informatics Education in Europe

Vol. 58. G. Riva, B.K. Wiederhold and E. Molinari (Eds.), Virtual Environments in Clinical Psychology and Neuroscience

Vol. 59. I.A.F. Stokes (Ed.), Research into Spinal Deformities 2

Vol. 60. M. Di Rienzo, G. Mancia, G. Parati, A. Pedotti and A. Zanchetti (Eds.), Methodology and Clinical Applications of Blood Pressure and Heart Rate Analysis

Vol. 61. R.A. Mortensen (Ed.), ICNP® and Telematic Applications for Nurses in Europe

Vol. 62. J.D. Westwood, H.M. Hoffman, R.A. Robb and D. Stredney (Eds.), Medicine Meets Virtual Reality

Vol. 63. R. Rogers and J. Reardon, Recommendations for International Action

Vol. 64. M. Nerlich and R. Kretschmer (Eds.), The Impact of Telemedicine on Health Care Management

Vol. 65. In production

Vol. 66. In production

ISSN: 0926-9630

Building Regional Health Care Networks in Europe

Edited by

John Oates

Sema Group, United Kingdom

Henrik Bjerregaard Jensen

The Danish Centre for Health Telematics, Denmark

Sponsored by

CENTIS
The Danish Centre for Health Telematics
Deutsche Telekom Berkom GmbH
Hospital de Móstoles
North Eastern Health Board
Olivetti Sanità spa
Sema Group UK Ltd
South and East Belfast Health and Social Services Trust

IOS
Press
Ohmsha

Amsterdam • Berlin • Oxford • Tokyo • Washington, DC

ISBN 0 9673355 9 0 (IOS Press)
ISBN 4 274 90325 7 C3047 (Ohmsha)
Library of Congress Catalog Card Number: 99-68223

Publisher
IOS Press
Van Diemenstraat 94
1013 CN Amsterdam
The Netherlands
fax: +31 20 620 3419
e-mail: order@iospress.nl

Distributor in the UK and Ireland
IOS Press/Lavis Marketing
73 Lime Walk
Headington
Oxford OX3 7AD
England
fax: +44 1865 75 0079

Distributor in the USA and Canada
IOS Press, Inc.
5795-G Burke Centre Parkway
Burke, VA 22015
USA
fax: +1 703 323 3668
e-mail: iosbooks@iospress.com

Distributor in Germany
IOS Press
Spandauer Strasse 2
D-10178 Berlin
Germany
fax: +49 30 242 3113

Distributor in Japan
Ohmsha, Ltd.
3-1 Kanda Nishiki-cho
Chiyoda-ku, Tokyo 101
Japan
fax: +81 3 3233 2426

Contents

INTRODUCTION	1
EXECUTIVE SUMMARY	3
1.VISION OF A COMPREHENSIVE RHCN	**8**
1.1 Health care is regional	**8**
1.2 Healthcare providers in a region	**8**
1.3 Information flows in regional health	**9**
1.3.1 Daily, routine information	9
1.3.2 Shared care information	10
1.3.3 Health information	10
1.3.4 Administrative information	11
1.4 The Regional Health Care Network - what is it?	**11**
1.5 RHCN - state of the art	**12**
1.5.1 National and European development	12
1.5.2 Barriers and lack of standard products	14
1.6 The RHCN - a vision	**15**
1.6.1 Breaking down barriers	15
1.6.2 The services in a future RHCN	16
1.6.3 Services and healthcare providers	20
1.6.4 Healthcare Telematic Services and the Internet	22
1.6.5 The regional Internet Node	23
1.7 Strategy: Building RHCNs in Europe	**25**
1.7.1 The overall strategy	25
1.7.2 Regional, national and European strategies needed	25
1.8 RHCNs - the impact and cost-benefits	**28**
2. RHCNs - MAKING IT HAPPEN	**31**
2.1 Framework Model for a successful RHCN strategy	**31**
2.1.1 Explanation of the Framework Model	31
2.1.2 Environment	34
2.1.3 Organisation, purpose and approach	42
2.1.4 Systems, processes and structure	50
2.1.5 Users	58
2.1.6 Partnerships	61
2.1.7 Resources	64

2.2 Risk factors and lessons learnt   69
  2.2.1 Risk factors   69
  2.2.2 Lessons learnt   71
  2.2.3 Do's and don'ts for implementing RHCNs   73

3. RHCNs - THE FUTURE (1998 - 2002)   75
  3.1 Products and services needed, 1998 - 2002   75
    3.1.1 Administrative transactions   76
    3.1.2 Booking service   77
    3.1.3 Clinical information   77
    3.1.4 Protocols and guidelines   79
    3.1.5 Multimedia information   79
  3.2 Industry and market trends - European and global   79
    3.2.1 Evolution of demand   79
    3.2.2 Products   80
    3.2.3 Market   81
    3.2.4 Comparison between EU and the rest of the world   84
  3.3 The need for standards   85
    3.3.1 The scenario   85
    3.3.2 The problems   86
    3.3.3 The goals   87
  3.4 Security - problems and solutions   88

4. RHCNs - A PERSPECTIVE BY COUNTRY   90
  4.1 European and global situation in RHCN   90
  4.2 National developments in RHCN, 1994 - 98   91
    4.2.1 Healthcare organisation   91
    4.2.2 Healthcare expenditure   93
    4.2.3 Information flows   93
    4.2.4 Service offerings   94
    4.2.5 Penetration of EHCRs   95
  4.3 Denmark   95
    4.3.1 Healthcare organisation   95
    4.3.2 Information flows   96
    4.3.3 IT systems in healthcare   97
    4.3.4 Current status of RHCN   98
    4.3.5 Industry - companies, products and services for RHCN   100
    4.3.6 Future development of RHCN, 1998 - 2002   100
  4.4 Finland   101
    4.4.1 Healthcare organisation   101

4.4.2 Information flows   102
4.4.3 IT systems in healthcare   102
4.4.4 Current status of RHCN   103
4.4.5 Industry - companies, products and services for RHCN   104
4.4.6 Future development of RHCN, 1998 - 2002   104
4.5 France   **104**
4.5.1 Healthcare organisation   104
4.5.2 Information flows   107
4.5.3 IT systems in healthcare   108
4.5.4 Current status of RHCN   110
4.5.5 Industry - companies, products and services for RHCN   111
4.5.6 Future development of RHCN, 1998 - 2002   112
4.6 Germany   **113**
4.6.1 Healthcare organisation   113
4.6.2 Information flows   114
4.6.3 IT systems in healthcare   115
4.6.4 Current status of RHCN   116
4.6.5 Industry - companies, products and services for RHCN   120
4.6.6 Future development of RHCN, 1998 - 2002   120
4.7 Ireland   **122**
4.7.1 Healthcare organisation   122
4.7.2 Information flows   123
4.7.3 IT systems in healthcare   124
4.7.4 Current status of RHCN   124
4.7.5 Industry - companies, products and services for RHCN   124
4.7.6 Future development of RHCN, 1998 - 2002   125
4.8 Italy   **125**
4.8.1 Healthcare organisation   125
4.8.2 Information flows   128
4.8.3 IT systems in healthcare   129
4.8.4 Current status of RHCN   131
4.8.5 Industry - companies, products and services for RHCN   132
4.8.6 Future development of RHCN, 1998 - 2002   133
4.9 Portugal   **135**
4.9.1 Healthcare organisation   135
4.9.2 Information flows   136
4.9.3 IT systems in healthcare   137
4.9.4 Current status of RHCN   138
4.9.5 Industry - companies, products and services for RHCN   139
4.9.6 Future development of RHCN, 1998 - 2002   140

4.10 Spain   140

    4.10.1 Healthcare organisation   140

    4.10.2 Information flows   141

    4.10.3 IT systems in healthcare   142

    4.10.4 Current status of RHCN   142

    4.10.5 Industry - companies, products and services for RHCN   142

    4.10.6 Future development of RHCN, 1998 - 2002   144

4.11 UK   146

    4.11.1 Healthcare organisation   146

    4.11.2 Information flows   148

    4.11.3 IT systems in healthcare   148

    4.11.4 Current status of RHCN   149

    4.11.5 Industry - companies, products and services for RHCN   150

    4.11.6 Future development of RHCN, 1998 - 2002   151

Appendix A: Glossary and Abbreviations   152

Appendix B: Healthcare Standardisation Organisations   157

Appendix C: References   167

Appendix D: Description of six EU IVFP projects building RHCNs   170

Authors/Contributors

Knut Bernstein, County of Funen – The Danish Centre for Health Telematics, Denmark
Leslie Boydell, South and East Belfast Health and Social Services Trust, UK
Carmen Ceinos, ECOMIT SL, Spain
Marco d'Angelantonio, HIM SA, Belgium
Nuno Estêvão, CENTIS S.A., Portugal
Bruno Frandji, SAPHIS, France
Edgar Glück, KITH (Norwegian Centre for Medical Informatics), Norway
Pentti Itkonen, North Karelia Hospital District, Finland
Henrik Bjerregaard Jensen, County of Funen – The Danish Centre for Health Telematics, Denmark
Santiago Marimon, CHC, Spain
John Oates, Sema Group, UK
Tony Reilly, North Eastern Health Board, Kells, Ireland
Dr Jan H. van Bemmel, The Netherlands
Mario Veloso, CENTIS S.A., Portugal
Andreas Weser, Deutsche Telekom Berkom GmbH, Germany
James Whannel, Systems Team Ltd, UK

Advisory Panel

Sune Andreasson, Project Manager in Stockholm, HSS
Pat Dolan, IT Manager, North Western Health Board, Ireland
Bob Ferguson, Chief Executive, South and East Belfast Health and Social Services Trust
Jose Maria de la Higuera, Director of Primary Care, Andalucia
Jaume Horrach, Hospital Manager, Balearic Islands
Pentti Itkonen, Director of Hospital District, Finland
Peder Jest, Medical Director, County of Funen, Denmark
Roberto Nardi, GP, SEMG representative, Italy
Sara Pupato, General Manager, Mostoles Hospital, Madrid
George Venters, Consultant in Public Health Medicine, Scotland

INTRODUCTION

Regional Health Care Networks (RHCN) are widely indicated as the natural evolution in the way healthcare is delivered.

Healthcare, over the last century, has undergone a revolution. From a situation where it was delivered by a single person, the family doctor, who knew everything about his patient and had a comprehensive understanding of the medical science and practice of his day, the healthcare delivery pattern has progressively moved towards a multitude of healthcare professionals having a specialist knowledge of an increasingly narrow field of medicine.

This has been an inevitable consequence of the incredible growth of medical knowledge, and of the increasing sophistication of diagnostic and therapeutic protocols, over a period of just a few decades. A single person, however knowledgeable, cannot master all the branches of modern medicine; healthcare professionals have evolved either towards the role of the General Practitioner (GP), understanding a little bit of everything, at least to the level of pointing his/her patient to the right specialist, or towards the role of a specialist with an in-depth training in just a single field of medicine.

Different types of healthcare professional tend to work in different settings; GPs are spread over the territory, close to the people in their place of residence, while specialists are grouped in a single place, the hospital or clinic, where dozens, hundreds and, sometimes, thousand of them are hosted in a single campus.

It is no wonder that the mentalities and practices of these two communities of healthcare professionals have grown apart over the years. Even communication between the two populations has become increasingly difficult because of different focus, pace, jargon etc. characterising one community versus the other. Lack of communication has led, in turn, to incomprehension between different communities of healthcare professionals and, in some cases, to mutual despite.

This lack of communication has certainly not benefited the patient, whose well being and health should have been the ultimate target of the healthcare system as a whole.

RHCNs are just about helping people, who have lost the habit of communicating with one another, to reopen the dialogue and start exchanging relevant clinical and managerial information to enable all health professionals to work better and to be more effective in their activity.

RHCNs are just a means, and can achieve results only where there is willingness among people to collaborate; playing with the words RHCN, i.e. telematics networks, help networks of people (the healthcare professionals) to work better for their clients, the patients.

RHCNs are good for Europe and for European citizens. They can also be good for the European industry if indigenous companies are able to capitalise on their current lead in this area, and play a dominant role in this market when it comes out of its infancy.

This Report is the fruit of a joint effort by a number of people who have been involved in the implementation of RHCNs throughout Europe in the last decade, brought together under the banner of a European project, WISE (Work in Synergy for Europe). We, because I myself am one of them, have made mistakes, and have suffered disappointments; but we have also enjoyed some remarkable successes. We have tried to build on our experience to distil the basic elements, which determine the success or failure of a RHCN.

We are strong believers in a bright future for RHCNs, and are so enthusiastic about their potential that most of us have already embarked on the next generation of projects under the 5th Framework Programme, to take RHCNs a few steps forwards. I hope that our enthusiasm will inspire those who have not yet entered this arena, and that they will be willing to follow us.

I hope that the reader will enjoy reading the Report, but even more I hope that he or she will find in here the answers to the many questions they might have about RHCNs and their implications.

On a personal note, I want to add that it has been a pleasure and an honour for me to co-ordinate the work of such a wonderful group of professionals, who have contributed to the production of this book, and that I am proud of the result that we have achieved.

Marco d'Angelantonio
WISE Project Co-ordinator

EXECUTIVE SUMMARY

Health care is regional.

Modern healthcare is not provided by one institution or by one group of healthcare professionals alone. Modern healthcare is provided in close co-operation between many different institutions and many different professional groups – working together and using their specialised expertise in their common effort to deliver the best quality service and most cost effective care as possible. Without this specialisation, it would not be possible to apply advanced techniques and the many distinct functions provided by hospitals, consultants, laboratories, nursing homes, social care etc.

Due to this specialisation and division of labour, the need for cross-sector information in healthcare is growing. The day-to-day communication between the different partners is vast, and crucial for cost, quality and service of the entire healthcare system. In the Netherlands, for example, 300 million clinical messages are exchanged annually between primary and secondary healthcare concerning individual patients' diagnoses and treatment. When adding to this the administration communications (which makes up about one-third of the medical data) the total amount of information exceeds the communication needs in, for example, the financial sector. In Denmark, the cost of communication between the different institutions in health is equal to 1 – 2% of total health expenditure.[1]

This cross-sector communication in healthcare is done manually today. The information is communicated using mail, phone, fax or carried by the patient – and the bulk of information is printed out from one IT system, mailed and finally re-keyed into another IT system used in another institution. This form of communication is costly, takes time and gives rise to failures.

Not surprisingly, several European investigations[2] have shown that lack of co-ordination and continuity in care is a main and growing problem in healthcare today.

Therefore the need for Regional Health Care Networks is obvious.

Regional networks make it possible to give healthcare providers access to the right information when they need it. Regional networks make it possible to exchange information more smoothly between different healthcare institutions and different healthcare professionals during the treatment of individual patients. Regional networks make it possible to guide the professionals, the patients and the public, to give better co-ordination and continuity in care.

Such Regional Health Care Networks should provide services for:
- Daily communication of prescriptions, lab-results etc.
- Secure e-mail systems for patient-related information.
- Booking-facilities for hospital and diagnostic services.
- Shared Medical records.
- Emergency and alert systems.
- Tele-medicine facilities.
- Protocols and guidelines for cross-sector treatment.

- Health Information web-sites to professionals, patients and the public.
- Administrative, cross-sector information and management systems.

Such comprehensive Regional Health Care Networks do not exist in Europe today.

However, in the last ten years several less comprehensive RHCNs have been developed on national and European initiatives. On national level, this started in UK and The Netherlands in the late eighties, with development of EDI links for communication between GPs and hospitals; it continued during the nineties in several European countries with focus areas other than GP-hospital links, and using a wide range of different communication technologies. In the same way, the European Telematic Application Programme for Health has funded large European projects working with research and development creating RHCNs.

Due to such activities, the political awareness for building RHCNs has risen significantly, and many regional and national healthcare authorities now have this topic as a part of their overall strategy for cross-sector co-operation in health.

But both national and European projects have meet barriers such as the lack of both European and national standards, the lack of common accepted clinical procedures, the unsolved contractual and legal issues, the high development costs, and the necessity of reaching a "critical mass" before regional services are useful.

Because of such barriers, the development of RHCNs in Europe is still only improving slowly. As a result of this, no off-the-shelf application products for RHCNs are available on the market. All the above mentioned national and European projects still mainly use proprietary and/or in-house IT solutions - a situation comparable to the situation for hospital IT systems at the beginning of the seventies.

Fortunately, however, the penetration of the Internet into society as a whole, and the experiences gained in the last 10 years, seem to make it possible to change this situation:

- First, the penetration of the Internet platform has created widespread consensus to use a single technological platform; this creates the possibility for industry to develop standard products with lower investments for a much larger market.

- Secondly, the experience gained from the national and European RHCN projects during the last ten years has made it possible to create a coherent and consistent vision of a comprehensive RHCN.

As described in section 1.6 The RHCN – a vision, it is likely that the standard Internet protocols will make it possible to fulfil most of the functionality needed in a comprehensive RHCN if the messaging and security technologies are combined with the Internet communication protocols; also as described in the same section, most of the functionality needed can be met by creating 18 types of standard services. This makes it possible for European industry to develop products and services as modules fitting into such a "standardised" comprehensive RHCN.

Table 1: Services in a comprehensive RHCN

RHCN Services		
Clinical Services	**Health Services**	**Administrative Services**
1. Clinical messages	9. Surveillance information	15. Reimbursement
2. Clinical e-mail	10. Yellow pages	16. Electronic commerce
3. Clinical booking	11. Professional guidelines	17. Patient-id
4. Shared records	12. Disease quality management	18. Resource management
5. Care protocols	13. Public health information	
6. Mobile and emergency	14. Continuing professional development	
7. Home-care monitoring		
8. Telemedicine		

To facilitate this process, public investment and a common strategy is necessary - on regional, national and European levels.

The aim of such a strategy is simple. By creating a common vision of the technique and services in a comprehensive future RHCN, it will become less risky for European industry to develop and market such IT solutions as standard products. But before being willing to invest significantly in the area, industry needs a commitment from healthcare authorities to work in the same direction. Therefore strategies for healthcare authorities on regional, national and European levels are needed to make it possible to adopt the vision.

The regional level

The most important players building RHCNs are the local regional healthcare authorities. In most European countries, these authorities are responsible for the co-ordination and continuity in the provision of healthcare services in the region. In many European countries, they are also directly responsible for delivering significant parts of the services in hospitals, home care units and other parts of the regional healthcare system.

To implement the RHCN in the region, the healthcare authority has to implement a regional Internet node. The regional node consists of one or more Internet Service Providers (ISPs) acting as entrusted third-parties for the regional healthcare authority providing the RHCN services to hospitals, GPs and home-care units on traditional commercial conditions.

Only a few of the 18 RHCN services could be provided from the beginning. On the contrary, most of the services demands significant organisational changes before being implemented; other services demand specific IT projects in the region. Therefore the regional healthcare authority has to develop a long-term strategy and business plan showing which RHCN services are going to be implemented, when and how. During this long term implementation process, the existing ways of cross-sector co-operation in the region have to be changed radically. Therefore building RHCNs in a region have to be a vital part of the health policy in the region, the part that copes with cross-sector co-ordination and cross-sector co-operation.

It is recommended that regional healthcare authorities:

- make long-term regional business plans and project organisation;
- certificate regional ISPs – and set up node with basic functionality;
- implement the RHCN services step by step – and adjust the organisation using adequate BPR processes.

The national level

Because of the barriers to building regional networks, a national strategy in this area is recommended, to co-ordinate and facilitate regional development and to secure cross-regional communication within the country. In some European countries, such national programmes have been started with significant influence on the regional implementation.

It is recommended that national authorities:

- create a national task-force to develop a RHCN strategy;
- develop national security rules and standards for communication;
- secure co-ordination between regional work, and support regional R&D.

The European level

Finally, a European initiative is needed to create a market for standard products for RHCN services.

European programmes for developing IT for healthcare have mostly been broad project calls making it possible to develop a wide range of services and products using a wide range of different technologies. However, as described above the main barrier to developing RHCNs on a large scale basis is the lack of standard industry products in the area; broad project calls are not helping the development of standard products.

Therefore, a more narrow programme is needed to fund and facilitate the development of the 18 RHCN services mentioned above on a common Internet platform. Such a narrow programme would make it more easy and less risky for European industry to focus their investment to specific, precise defined services for RHCN, and would be a major driving force creating widespread consensus on the content of the services needed.

Such a dedicated programme could be a natural part of the overall European Information Society Telematic (IST) programme which is aimed at developing the same lines as described in this vision of building RHCNs. Together with the development of the regional and national strategies, this could create a platform for a coherent, firm and co-ordinated strategy, which would ensure large scale development of RHCNs in Europe, and result in standard industry products.

At the European level, it is recommended:

- to develop a narrow IST programme supporting regions implementing the services described;
- to strengthen the European work developing standards for communication.

This book has been written in co-operation between the European Commission, and the six European projects in the IVth Framework Programme aimed at RHCN problems: CHIN, CoCo, Ithaca, Prestige, REMEDES and Star. These projects have in the period 1995 – 1998 gained significant experience by piloting RHCN services in 45 different regions in 14 European countries; hundreds of healthcare professionals have been involved.

This book gathers the experiences, the opportunities and the failures made by the projects, and presents the state-of-the-art in the area.

But, building on ten years of experience in creating RHCNs in Europe, this book also presents a proposal for a vision and a strategy for building large scale RHCNs in Europe.

CHAPTER 1

1.   VISION OF A COMPREHENSIVE RHCN

1.1   Health care is regional

In the last twenty years, the provision of health services has changed from having GP and general hospitals as the main focus of healthcare, towards a health system with a range of different specialised functions co-operating in the provision of care.

These developments are reflected in the administrative organisation of health care[a]. In Italy, for example, a health reform in the nineties created 223 Local Health Authorities (USLs), typically covering about 300.000 inhabitants. The Local Health Authorities are responsible for hospitals and community care, together with independent hospitals and independent GPs and Free Choice Paediatricians. In Scandinavia, UK and Ireland, healthcare has traditionally been organised around regions.

In some European countries, however, the regional structure is not so clear. In Germany, the key-stone for healthcare provision is a complex public and private insurance system – in principle a national system. In practice, however, the patients and professionals have a more restricted range for choosing healthcare services.

A health region is the geographical area where most health services are provided to the inhabitants in the area, and in which area the patient typically receives almost all of the health services they need. In many healthcare regions, the population is around 0,5 million, unless in large cities, where the "natural" healthcare region normally covers the whole city, and can therefore grow to many million inhabitants.

1.2   Healthcare providers in a region

The most important healthcare providers in a region are:

1. Primary care providers such as GPs or local health centres.
2. Pharmacies.
3. Laboratories and other diagnostic centres used by both primary and secondary care.
4. Secondary hospitals.
5. Tertiary, specialised hospital.
6. Specialists or consultants.
7. Other health providers like dentists, physiotherapist and chiropractic clinics.
8. Home care providers and midwife services.

Beside these regional providers, a range of expert services are provided nationally; typically these are hospitals which act as "centres of excellence" for specific diseases, and highly specialised laboratories and other diagnostic expert centres.

---

a   The organisation of healthcare in different European countries is described in chapter 4.

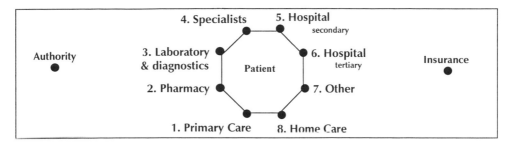

Figure 1: Regional Healthcare Providers

In the administrative area, the organisation differs more; this tends to depend on the degree to which healthcare services are paid by insurance (which is typically delivered nationally) or public paid (which is typically delivered regionally).

The administrative partners are typically:
- national, private or public insurance companies;
- national, regional or local healthcare authorities.

1.3   Information flows in regional health

The information flows in a healthcare region can be divided in four groups:
- daily, routine information;
- shared care information;
- health information;
- administrative information.

1.3.1   Daily, routine information

The most important and most frequent communication flows in regional healthcare are the direct result of specialisation occurring when one healthcare provider orders a service from another provider, and afterwards receives the result. This patient-related information is well known in all European countries, and consists of information such as prescriptions, laboratory requests and results, referrals, discharge information, and other information resulting from ordering services as a part of the diagnosis and treatment of the individual patient – the patient-related information. This information is very frequent; investigations from Denmark[3,4] have shown that 1–2% of the total resources in healthcare are used to communicate about 40 million messages annually between the parties in healthcare provision.

Due to its purpose, this "order-result" communication is normally form-based, short and textual – and transferred by mail, phone, fax or carried by the patient herself. For the same reasons, it is possible to communicate such information electronically using quite "old-fashioned" technology such as normal phone lines, modems and store-and-forward techniques. On the other hand, this routine communication is so frequent that it is driving the need for structured communication, which makes possible integration between the IT applications already in use by the healthcare professionals.

In recent years, there has been political awareness in several European countries of a more modern and service oriented way of ordering services in health care - a demand for "booking-facilities" as known from travel and flight services. This new type of communication substitutes some of the order-result communication mentioned above, especially when the patient is directly involved.

There is therefore a need for services in RHCNs making it possible to:
- communicate daily, routine information as structured, standardised messages or as unstructured text using cheap but secured e-mail;
- make on-line cross-sector booking of treatment and investigations.

1.3.2   Shared care information

The other patient-related type of information flow in regional healthcare is the second most important, but not at all so frequently used as the daily, routine messages. Shared care information is needed in situations where several healthcare institutions are participating in the treatment of the same groups of patients. For example, in the treatment of diabetic patients[5], hospitals, GPs and home care are normally involved, and optimal care is dependent on adequate information and co-ordination between these three healthcare providers. Another example is the treatment of elderly people, who often need intervention from GPs and home care after hospitalisation.

Surprisingly, formal co-ordination of the care of such groups of patients is often very poor, or even non-existent. There is therefore a growing interest in developing cross-sector care protocols for specific group of patients; this normally results in significant improvements in quality and service, together with a reduction of costs.

Finally, the development of new IT technologies has put focus on the opportunities to provide care to remote patients situated in isolated areas without adequate professional expertise or equipment. Modern telecommunication facilities make it possible to provide "tele-consultation" from experts to other health professionals situated far from the experts, and "tele-monitoring" of patients at home. Also, the possibility of formalising "second opinion" from colleagues could improve quality of care.

There is therefore a need for services in RHCNs making it possible to:
- share patient records between different healthcare providers;
- exchange specific defined health data as a part of care protocol guided treatment;
- have on-line, multimedia access between health professionals for tele-consultation, tele-monitoring, or assistance to emergency units and mobile home-care professionals.

1.3.3   Health information

In healthcare, there has for many years been a tradition of producing written guidelines and catalogues with health information for professionals or for patients. Such types of information do not contain information about individual patients, but consists of general information about how to treat patients with specific diseases, information on specific types of healthcare providers, and guidelines for health education for the public in general.

The new technologies, especially Internet, make it possible to communicate such general health information much more effectively and to reach many new groups of users. There are plenty of examples of the need for such general health information databases, such as "yellow pages" with practical information (name, address, phone, employees, services etc) from the healthcare providers in the regions, guidelines for the treatment of special diseases in hospitals, general regional rules for referral of patients to other health providers, and health promotion information to the public in general or to specific patient groups.

There is therefore a need for services in RHCNs making it possible to give access to:
- the general public, to updated yellow pages about regional health providers;
- health professionals, to standard procedures and referral rules;
- health professionals, for cross-sector disease quality management.

1.3.4   Administrative information

Finally in healthcare, as in other sectors, much communication is covering the need for administration, finance and management purposes. Because healthcare in most countries is the largest sector, ranging from 6 to 10 % of the GNP, the administrative communication is vast. In contrast to the clinical information, the administrative information differs from country to country, due to differences in organisation and the degree of public and private payment. Nevertheless, reimbursement is a main task in healthcare in all European countries, and so is the need for professionals to make an exact and quick identification of patients. As a result of the growing liberalisation in health in many European countries, the need for regional resource management information in relation to demand and supply of health services is growing.

There is therefore a need for services in RHCNs making it possible to:
- reimburse for provided health services to public and private insurance;
- order and pay for goods and services using tools for electronic commerce;
- have easy access to patient-ID systems;
- have overall management information making rational and effective resource management possible.

1.4   The Regional Health Care Network - what is it?

Following the above-mentioned need, it is possible to set up a common definition of a Regional Health Care Network:

"The RHCN connects the different healthcare providers in the region, making it possible to access and exchange information electronically between hospitals, GPs, patients, health centres, laboratories and other healthcare institutions in the region."

RHCN makes secure information sharing and secure communication between healthcare providers and patients possible using regional telematic systems to provide co-ordinated patient care. The communication could be structured or unstructured, textual or multimedia, integrated or stand-alone, depending on the actual needs and the organisational, financial and technological opportunities.

- Using a RHCN, the healthcare professionals should have the opportunity to access data about a specific patient from many different places at any time, regardless of which institution the patient is being treated in for the moment.

- Using a RHCN, it should be possible to transfer automatically, correctly and immediately clinical and administrative information between hospitals, GPs, laboratories, ambulances, insurance companies and to the patient's home, creating seamless and cost-effective care despite the fact that many different providers are involved.

- Using a RHCN, it should be possible to integrate healthcare systems used by different healthcare institutions, in such a way that the end-user does not need to be concerned with different databases or formats, and can easily access the information needed to provide care for the patient.

- Using a RHCN, it should be possible for patients and citizens to get access to health information and health provision in the region.

1.5   RHCN – state of the art

1.5.1   National and European development

Since the beginning of the nineties, there have been research and development activities on RHCNs at regional, national and European level, a few at the beginning of the decade, and several in the last five years. These activities have resulted in pilot projects and operational RHCNs in several European regions; these are all quite different in scale, provide different services, and have different regional healthcare providers participating.

The development of RHCNs started in UK; as a result of the "Working for Patient" reform in the beginning of the nineties, a national healthcare network infrastructure was created, with EDI standards. An effort also started in the Netherlands and Scandinavia, and resulting in operational RHCNs focussing on messaging between GPs, hospitals and health authorities.

In the last part of the decade, most other European countries have started building RHCNs using different types of technology, and a broader approach to RHCNs than just messaging. In Ireland, Finland, Italy, Spain, France, Portugal and Belgium, building RHCNs is now more or less a part of the health authorities policy for developing IT in health care; but all projects in all countries are still meeting severe barriers to reach large scale use.

The development and current state of RHCNs around Europe are discussed in chapter 4, but Table 2 below identifies a number of such networks.

Besides national developments, the European Commission have been supporting IT development through the TAP programme for research and development of telematic applications for health. In the IVth Framework Programme (running 1995 – 98), six projects have been working on building RHCNs; the total investment has been 30.8 million euros; with funding from the EU totalling 14.9 million euros.

Table 2: Regional Health Care Networks in Europe, 1998

ALDABIDE	Intranet, voice and management systems in Basque Region. 1997. Spain.
Catalan Health Service	Internet and e-mail network in Catalan region.1997. Spain.
CHIN	Regional intranet with patient records and telemedicine. 1998.
CoCo	Regional EDI networks for GPs in several regions. 1998.
CUP2000	Booking-system and laboratory result in city of Bologna. 1998. Italy.
DGN	National network for Internet-access, databases and banking. 1998. Germany.
GHC	National network WEB-access, e-mail and medical databases.1999. Germany.
GPS	National reimbursement of prescriptions. 1999. Ireland.
INSEIL	Health-net in Friuli-Venezia-Guilia region. 1996. Italy.
Ithaca	System for shared care for elderly people. 1998.
KV	National network for reimbursement for GPs. 1994. Germany.
MedCom	National EDI network for primary care. 1994. Denmark.
NHSnet	National network for linking all health service organisations. 1995. UK.
NWHB	GP-links to Hospitals in NWHB. 1997. Ireland.
Prestige	System for clinical protocols and guidelines. 1998.
Racal Healthlink	National network for GP to Health Authority links. 1990. UK.
REMEDES	Booking, mail and request/result system. 1997.
RIS	Connection between healthcare regions. 1998. Portugal.
SIS	Health care net in Lombard-region. 1999. Italy.
STAR	Yellow Pages, Patient-ID and booking applications. 1998.
VHN	Regional purchases system. 1997. Valencia Spain.

The six projects are:

- **The CHIN project** develops regional health care networks building on Internet technologies, and focusing on shared patient records and telemedicine between the healthcare providers. The CHIN project is piloted in Berlin, Scotland, Umeå, Norrland (Sweden), North Karelia (Finland), Barcelona and Athens/Lavrion.
- **The CoCo project** develops regional health care networks building on VANS technologies, and focusing on standardisation of messages (EDI) of discharge notes, referrals, prescriptions etc. between GPs, hospitals, pharmacies and home care. The CoCo-project is piloted in Funen, Belfast, NW Ireland, Barcelona, Manacor, West Norway, Rhodes, Zwolle, Bergamo and Ipswich.
- **The ITHACA project** develops regional health care building on a shared medical record using client-server applications, and focusing on shared care between hospitals and community care for elderly, maternity, child care, and mental illness groups. The Ithaca project is piloted in Belfast, Andalucia, Turku, Porto, Oise, Bergamo, Amaroussion, Gothenburg, Dublin, Cavan and Saskatchewan.
- **The Prestige project** develops regional health care networks building on client-server techniques, and focusing on clinical protocols and guidelines for quality improvement of the treatment of specific patient groups cared for in co-operation between hospitals

and GPs. The Prestige project is piloted in Lisboa valley, Tejo, Modena, Funen, London, Mainz and Eaton.

- **The REMEDES project** develops regional health care networks building on client-server applications, and focusing on booking, electronic mail and laboratory request and result communication between GPs and hospitals. The Remedes project is piloted in Bergamo, Montpellier, Cambridge & Huntingdon, Madrid and Manacor (Belearics).
- **The STAR project** develops regional health care networks building on the Internet technology, and focusing on booking, yellow pages functions and central patient-id facilities in a RHCN covering many different providers in a region. The Star project is piloted in NE Ireland, Stockholm, Milan, Crete, Delft, Helsinki, Middlesex and Basque.

The European projects are described in detail in Appendix D.

As can be seen from the description above, the ongoing research and development has been growing steadily in the last 10 years. Today, all European countries and most of the different types of healthcare providers are involved; they are focusing on many different types of services for regional health. Looking at the efforts made by the European Commission, the six EU projects mentioned above have gathered experience from as much as 45 different pilot projects in 14 countries covering hundreds of hospitals, GPs, home care units and involving 32 different healthcare authorities. Altogether, this mean that Europe are now the world leaders in building RHCNs - in close competition with the USA.

1.5.2 Barriers and lack of standard products

Despite the fact of growing political awareness, severe barriers still exist before a self-sustained market can develop. These barriers are well known when implementing IT systems in a fragmented healthcare sector, but are even more of an issue when coping with regional IT systems involving many different and independent organisations and providers.

These barriers are created by failures in the following areas:
- long term visions for co-ordination, continuity and cross-sector co-operation;
- political leadership and defined responsibilities for "the region";
- agreement on dividing costs and benefits when introducing cross-sector IT systems;
- support from professionals for organisational change and cross-sector co-operation, in particular between the health and social sectors;
- common standards, protocols, guidelines, terminology and agreement of security rules;
- documented costs and benefits for regional IT systems;
- formulated strategies at regional, national and European level;
- established partnerships between industry, authorities and professionals.

But the most important barrier is the lack of standard products. All the above-mentioned regional, national and European projects and programmes have to a large degree developed bespoke (i.e. specifically developed) RHCN services for local use, in the same way as was done for IT solutions to hospitals and laboratories in the beginning of the seventies. In other words, mass-market products are still absent in the area of RHCNs; developments are therefore costly and slow.

One of the reasons for this lack of standard products is an unclear and confused common understanding of a RHCN, and the functionality needed for the IT services in RHCNs.

This lack of industry applications has to be filled before RHCNs can develop on a large scale in Europe. In this way, the situation for RHCNs is very similar to the situation of IT in health in general in the beginning of the seventies.

This situation can only be solved by central initiatives – initiatives from regional, national and European authorities building on a common and agreed strategy.

Fortunately, however, the experiences from the last 10 years of research and development in RHCNs, together with the rapid penetration of Internet into society in the last few years, seem to make it possible to change this situation in the future:

- Using the experiences of the ongoing RHCN projects it is now possible to make an overall description of the needs and services in a comprehensive RHCN, making it possible for industry to focus their investment on specific defined areas of need – and providing solutions for a European market.

- Due to the penetration of the Internet platform in Europe as a whole, it is now possible to chose a common technological platform for all services which reduces investment and risks significantly; this therefore makes affordable products a realistic possibility.

- Due to the widespread political awareness by regional and national authorities and in the European Commission, it is now possible to set up a common strategy for building regional health care networks on a large scale in Europe.

In the following section, a proposal for a vision of the future RHCN and a common strategy will be outlined.

1.6   The RHCN – a vision

1.6.1   Breaking down barriers

As described above, the RHCNs in Europe are today building on bespoke IT solutions made by local IT industry in the various regions. This situation results in high costs for the regional healthcare providers, and makes large scale development of RHCNs in Europe impossible.

But because of ten years of experience building RHCNs in Europe, and because of the penetration of the Internet, it is now possible to make a qualified proposal for the most important services in a comprehensive RHCN, all using the same technological platform. Such a strategy would make it less risky for the industry to provide products, and at the same time the RHCN becomes more affordable for the healthcare authorities.

The vision of a future RHCN:

- describes 18 main services needed in a comprehensive RHCN, which could be developed and implemented step-by-step in the region following the local health strategy for cross-sector co-operation;

- builds on a regional Internet node established in the region consisting of one or more Internet Services Providers (ISP's) which are acting as a trusted third party for the regional healthcare authorities.

1.6.2   The services in a future RHCN

The Services provided in a comprehensive RHCN cover Clinical Services, Health Services and Administrative Services.

Table 3: Services in a comprehensive RHCN

RHCN Services		
Clinical Services	**Health Services**	**Administrative Services**
1. Clinical messages	9. Surveillance information	15. Reimbursement
2. Clinical e-mail	10. Yellow pages	16. Electronic commerce
3. Clinical booking	11. Professional guidelines	17. Patient-id
4. Shared records	12. Disease quality management	18. Resource management
5. Care protocols	13. Public health information	
6. Mobile and emergency	14. Continuing professional development	
7. Home-care monitoring		
8. Telemedicine		

- Clinical Services are patient-related information to healthcare professionals used during the care of the individual patient.

- Health Services provide health-related information to the general public, to specific groups of patients, or to health professionals. These services do not contain patient-related information.

- Administrative Services are information to professionals to be used for administration and management issues.

1.6.2.1 Clinical Services

The Clinical Services are the most important functionality in a RHCN, and consist of patient-related information concerning the treatment of the individual patient.

1. **Clinical Messages** is a service making it possible to exchange form-based information such as prescriptions, laboratory results, referrals and discharge summaries almost automatically between different providers of health. When communicating Clinical Messages, a "store and forward" e-mail technique is often used because of the well known technique and the opportunity to communicate 24 hours/day. Because such messaging is suitable for standardisation, national or regional standards make it possible to integrate Clinical Messages in IT applications already in use by the professionals in the region. This is done to varying extents today in UK, The Netherlands and Scandinavia, where EDI standards cover the most

frequent messages in primary healthcare; this approach has also been dominant in the EU CoCo project.

Examples: Prescriptions, results and requests for laboratory, radiology, MRI, ultrasound and ECG services, referrals, discharge summaries, medical record, client history, intervention etc.

2. **Clinical e-mail** is a secure, firewall-protected and/or encrypted e-mail service dedicated to transfer patient-related information. Today telephones are used very frequently to give short, but important, patient-related information; normal e-mail would be very adequate to use in these cases. Nevertheless, e-mail is not used much for cross-sector communication, among other reasons because of the need for special security in health. In Germany, Norway and UK, the authorities are working on guidelines for security in this area.

    Examples: All unstructured textual e-mail messages and attachments (text, pictures, figures) transferring patient-related information between different healthcare professionals.

3. **Clinical Booking** is an IT service making it possible to book an appointment for treatment or investigation at other hospitals or specialist clinics. In Clinical Booking, an immediate answer is needed, and therefore on-line IT systems are normally used. Due to political awareness in Italy and Spain, booking services are actually provided in these countries; Clinical Booking is a main topic in the EU Remedes project.

    Examples: During the consultation at the GP, an appointment for investigation in a radiology clinic is made, making it possible for the patient to chose between several dates for the investigation. The ideal situation could be illustrated from travel agencies, where the customers have access to a complete catalogue of everything provided, and are able from this to book a trip taking costs, quality and date into account.

4. **Shared Record** is an IT service making it possible to share patient record data for the same patient between different professionals in different institutions in the region. Record Sharing demands a high degree of functionality and common structure, and such services therefore often use the same IT application, distributed to different professionals.

    Examples: In the EU Ithaca project, such cross-sector medical systems were developed for three patient groups: the elderly, children and disabled people.

5. **Care Protocols** is an IT service making it possible to transfer exact defined information between health professionals in cases where different professionals participate in the treatment of the same patient group. Before communication is possible, protocols and guidelines have to be defined and agreed by the participating professionals, stating who should provide what treatment. The EU Prestige project has care protocols as its main focus.

    Examples: Transferring specific datasets between hospitals, midwifes, GPs and community care in connection to births. Transferring specific datasets from outpatient clinic to GPs and community care following a common agreed protocol in which the division of labour and guidelines for the treatment are described.

6.   **Mobile & Emergency** are IT services dedicated to support mobile units like ambulances, doctors on duty and home nurses visiting patients at home. It makes it possible to transfer patient related information from systems at home-care units and in GP surgeries, in order to get access to the patient's journal and retrieve updated information or save new information.

      Examples: On-line access to the healthcare record held by the GP when visiting the patient at home, and transferring updated information on changes in medication after the visit. Another example is providing expert supervision to ambulance staff in pre-hospital emergency situations.

7.   **Home-Care Monitoring** is an IT service making it possible to look after patients located at home, often as alert systems making it possible for weak patients to call assistance.

      Examples: To keep elderly patients in their own home as long as possible, it is necessary to set up alert systems to call doctors or nurses in situations where the patient is getting worse. Such systems could either be automatically activated, or manually by the patient him/herself, and could result in a visit by the home nurse, or an emergency alarm or voice contact to a central unit.

8.   **Telemedicine** is an IT service used during the actual care of patients, making it possible to provide expert supervision to other professionals or directly to the patient. Telemedicine is the "classic" health telematic service, and is especially relevant if large geographic distances are a problem. In Norway, Scotland and France, there have been significant initiatives in this area for several years.

      Examples: On-line video conference or tele-consultation from remote experts during the actual investigation or treatment of a patient. Tele-monitoring of a patient situated alone at home or transferring an alert from a device on the client's body.

1.6.2.2 Health Services

Health Services are information services providing health-related information to the public in general, to specific patient groups, or to specific groups of healthcare professionals. The information is typically general guidelines and procedures, and not information about the individual patient. The main types are yellow pages, guidelines for healthcare professionals, disease quality management and public health information.

9.   **Surveillance Information** are IT systems dedicated to communicate epidemiological information to professionals for medical surveillance. Such information are today typically gathered by national research-institutes and distributed regularly by means of newsletters etc.

10.   **Yellow Pages** is an IT service making it possible to get practical information about healthcare providers, often with advanced facilities to search data in large databases.

The Internet-based Web sites technology has in recent years resulted in the appearance of many such yellow pages from hospitals, health authorities etc.

Examples: Addresses, phone numbers, hospital services, names of employees etc.

11. **Professional guidelines** are services for healthcare professionals with general information and guidelines about cost, quality, protocols and procedures, making it possible for health professionals to improve their practice. The gate-keeper role of GPs in many European countries especially has crystallised the need for such information systems.

    Examples: Information to GPs about cost, quality and waiting times for hospital treatment in different hospitals in the region.

12. **Disease Quality Management** are services with information making it possible for health professionals to optimise care quality when making cross sector treatment of specific diagnoses.

    Examples: Standardised reporting to a regional database of quality parameters for treatment of special groups of patients, making it possible for each health provider to compare their own and other providers' results in order to improve their individual treatment.

13. **Public Health Information** is a service to the public in general or to specific patient groups to inform and guide about diseases, prevention and services provided by the regional healthcare system.

    Examples: Web-based information provided by hospitals, patient associations and counties to inform and guide patients how to use the health system.

14. **Continuing Professional Development** is a service to the healthcare professionals, to make it possible to improve their education continuously.

    Examples: Medical expert-systems tutoring doctors in different and difficult diagnostic situations; news groups on the Internet are already frequently used for CPD in specific areas.

1.6.2.3 Administrative Services

Administrative Services are regional health services to professionals related to administrative, financial and management issues in health. The most well known services are reimbursement, electronic commerce, central patient-ID databases and regional resource management systems.

15. **Reimbursement** is a service making it possible to transfer bills from healthcare professionals to public or private insurance. Despite the fact that healthcare organisation differs between the countries in Europe, the reimbursement situation is important in all countries and is often the first regional telematic implementation in health. In Switzerland and Germany, electronic reimbursement is functioning on a large scale for many health professionals.

Examples: Transfer of reimbursement data from GPs to insurance companies, typically using national EDI standards.

16. **Electronic Commerce** is an IT-service making it possible to order, deliver and pay for goods and services to healthcare. In trade, the UN EDIFACT standards are used world-wide for this purpose; the developments are supported by the international EDIFACT and EAN organisations.

   Examples: Pharmacies ordering of drugs.

17. **Patient-id** is an IT service making it possible for health professionals to access central databases for quick and secure identification of patients. Because of lack of well known national ID-numbers, a secure identification of patients is a problem in several countries.

   Examples: National patient-ID databases in UK and Portugal.

18. **Resource management** are IT services providing information to health professionals giving access to cost and quality information from other health providers in the region. Especially in countries which have introduced provider-purchaser systems in health, where knowledge of costs and quality has become important for healthcare professionals and administrators.

   Examples: Web sites providing comparable information on costs and quality in order to make contracts between health buyers and health purchasers.

1.6.3 Services and healthcare providers

Not all services are used by all regional healthcare providers; on the contrary, some services are much more relevant for the co-operation between some providers than others. In Table 4 below, the main users of the different healthcare services are shown, together with an indication of which RHCN services are most relevant for each type of user.

Table 4: Main users of the RHCN services

	1. Primary Care	2. Pharmacies	3. Laboratories diagnostics	4. Specialists	5. Secondary Hospital	6. Tertiary Hospital	7. Other providers	8. Home Care	9. Authorities	10. Insurance	11. Patients
1. Clinical messages	✓	✓	✓	✓	✓		✓	✓			
2. Clinical e-mail	✓	✓	✓	✓	✓		✓	✓			
3. Clinical booking	✓		✓	✓	✓		✓				✓
4. Shared records	✓	✓		✓	✓	✓	✓	✓			
5. Care protocols	✓	✓		✓	✓	✓	✓	✓		✓	✓
6. Mobile & emergency	✓				✓	✓	✓	✓			
7. Home-care monitoring	✓				✓		✓	✓			✓
8. Telemedicine	✓			✓	✓	✓	✓				✓

	1. Primary Care	2. Pharmacies	3. Laboratories diagnostics	4. Specialists	5. Secondary Hospital	6. Tertiary Hospital	7. Other providers	8. Home Care	9. Authorities	10. Insurance	11. Patients
9. Surveillance information	✓			✓	✓	✓	✓		✓		
10. Yellow pages	✓			✓	✓	✓	✓		✓	✓	
11. Professional guidelines	✓	✓	✓	✓	✓	✓	✓	✓	✓		
12. Disease quality management	✓				✓	✓			✓		
13. Public health information											✓
14. Continuing professional development	✓	✓	✓	✓	✓	✓	✓				
15. Reimbursement	✓	✓	✓	✓			✓			✓	
16. Electronic commerce		✓	✓	✓	✓	✓	✓			✓	
17. Patient-id	✓	✓	✓	✓	✓	✓	✓		✓	✓	
18. Resource management	✓				✓	✓	✓	✓		✓	

In the same way, not all RHCN services are equally important and relevant to different providers. Some services cover a very broad group of healthcare activities in many types of institutions; some services are more relevant for special treatments, maybe not occurring very often. For example, daily, routine information is vital for most healthcare institutions and most healthcare professionals, and is needed many times each day. On the other hand, some RHCN services are only used on special occasions, for example tele-consultations from specialised health professionals in tertiary hospitals to remotely situated GPs in catastrophe situations. Nevertheless, most people would expect that it is also important to cover these unusual situations with adequate IT services.

Table 5 below shows the main possibilities for improving health for each of the services provided in RHCNs. All services could be used as tools for improving all types of benefits, but those identified are especially relevant .

Table 5: Main benefits of RHCN service

	Net savings	Improving quality of treatment	Improving services of professionals	Improving continuity of care	Improving service to patients
1. Clinical messages			++	++	
2. Clinical e-mail	✓		✓		
3. Clinical booking				✓	✓
4. Shared records		✓	✓	✓	
5. Care protocols		✓		✓	
6. Mobile & emergency		✓			
7. Home-care monitoring		✓			✓
8. Telemedicine		✓	✓		

	Net savings	Improving quality of treatment	Improving services of professionals	Improving continuity of care	Improving service to patients
9. Surveillance information			✓		
10. Yellow pages			✓		✓
11. Professional guidelines		✓	✓		
12. Disease quality management		✓	✓		
13. Public health information			✓		✓
14. Continuing professional development		✓	✓		✓
15. Reimbursement	✓				
16. Electronic commerce	✓				
17. Patient-id		✓	✓		
18. Resource management	✓				

1.6.4   Healthcare Telematic Services and the Internet

In line with the general acceptance and use of the Internet, the main services, "mail" and "web", are increasingly used by healthcare professionals to support various working scenarios.

The store-and-forward transmission characteristic of Internet mail, which makes it possible to communicate e-mail, and attach files, pictures, voice and video sequences in a very easy way, and the security mechanisms available often meet the practical needs for communication of:

- EDI messages of cross-sector daily, routine information, replacing some of the present use of forms;
- secure e-mail of cross-sector daily, routine information replacing some of the present use of phone and fax;
- care protocols with pre-defined cross-sector information between providers treating the same group of patients;
- tele-medicine with the attachment of pictures, video and graphics between GPs and specialists;
- reimbursement using pre-defined EDI standards to ensure compatibility;
- electronic commerce using standards for ordering and payment.

The Internet web service has proved to be an efficient means to communicate information such as:

- professional guidelines;
- information on disease quality management;
- epidemiology surveillance;
- clinical protocols;
- public health information to inform patient groups and the public in general.

In addition, web based distributed applications are going to significantly meet the needs e.g. for:

- healthcare resource management: e.g. booking applications, making on-line cross-sector booking possible from GPs to hospitals;
- virtual integration of patient records: cross-sector shared record systems where different providers are participating in the treatment and care of the same patients.

Hence, many of the described needs for cross-sector communication in regional health can be fulfilled by combining EDI and security techniques with the standard Internet protocols. The following table summarises some of the essential communication scenarios. Clinical mail and messaging is of particular relevance for medical emergency services. All scenarios can be implemented not only on the basis of terrestrial communication networks but also using wireless networks to support mobile users, for example using notebook PC or personal digital assistants. Of course, restrictions in the performance of end-user systems, graphical display characteristics and bandwidths have to be taken into account.

Table 6: Internet protocols and RHCN services

	1. Secure Mail	2. WEB pages	3. WEB applications
1. Clinical messages	✓		
2. Clinical e-mail	✓		
3. Clinical booking			✓
4. Shared records			✓
5. Care protocols	✓		✓
6. Mobile & emergency			✓
7. Home-care monitoring	✓		✓
8. Telemedicine	✓		✓
9. Surveillance information		✓✓	
10. Yellow pages		✓✓	
11. Professional guidelines		✓✓	✓
12. Disease quality management		✓✓	✓
13. Public health information		✓✓	
14. Continuing professional development		✓	✓
15. Reimbursement	✓✓		
16. Electronic commerce	✓		
17. Patient-id			✓
18. Resource management			✓

1.6.5   The regional Internet Node

As mentioned earlier, the existing research and development projects have used different platforms, depending on the technology available when they were planned: mainframe, client-server and VANS technology.

However, it is likely that in the future it will be possible to fulfil the main needs for RHCN services by integrating EDI techniques and security techniques in the general Internet platform:

- **EDI techniques**, in order to make it possible to exchange standardised messages automatically between the legacy IT systems used by the healthcare providers in the region.

- **Security techniques**, for encryption and/or firewall, to change the open Internet to a closed intranet so that patient-related information can be exchanged under secure conditions.

The Regional Node

The Regional Node is one or several ISPs who provide RHCN services to professionals in hospitals, GP surgeries, laboratories, home-care units etc.

The Regional Node has to be secured by a common firewall, and/or a common system of encryption has to be established, to make it possible for all healthcare professionals to get access to all other healthcare professionals – independent of which ISP the user has chosen.

In order to create competition in the RHCN, several independent, but connected, ISPs could be chosen by the regional health authority as nodes. In this case, a certification process is needed to secure 24 hour access for agreed services, common support arrangements, minimum performance requirements etc.

From the beginning the Regional Node has to implement these facilities:
- an RHCN portal showing the services available in the region;
- a key-centre providing keys and passwords because of the firewall and encryption process;
- a support centre making it possible to guide the users and track missing information;
- a yellow page system showing which healthcare providers are using what types of RHCN services, and the practical information to communicate (name, phone, e-mail address, IP-address, medical conditions for communication etc.);
- a patient-id service securing a regional (or national) 1-1 identification of patients.

When the regional authority has established this infrastructure, it is possible for the healthcare providers to join the RHCN, in the same way as joining any other Internet Service Provider.

The remaining services can then be implemented step-by-step, following the health policy in the region. They are described above in section 1.6.2.

1.7   Strategy: Building RHCNs in Europe

1.7.1   The overall strategy

The main barrier to large scale implementation is the lack of standard industry products provided for a European market for RHCNs.

All the RHCNs projects and programmes have so far mainly used local bespoke IT solutions, making the development costly and slow, and making it impossible to exploit the solutions on a large scale.

Fortunately, however, the research and development in the last 10 years has now made it possible to set up a vision of a future comprehensive RHCN building on standard industry products.

The main services which have to be developed to fulfil the needs are those described in section 1.6. Most of these services have been piloted in one or more of the 45 pilots participating in one of the six EU projects, described in Appendix D, in the IVth Framework TAP Programme. However, this does not mean that the products and services are ready for the European market. Most of the services are still on a research and development level. The services are also developed on different technological platforms due to historical and local reasons.

The penetration of the internet technologies has now made it possible to obtain consensus for one single technological platform for all the mentioned services. As described in section 1.6, it is likely that the standard facilities in the Internet makes it possible to fulfil most of the functionality needed in a comprehensive RHCN, provided that the EDI and security technologies are combined with the Internet communication protocols.

This networks will not be built by the market alone. Due to a lot of different barriers, central initiatives and investments are needed, in the same way that central investment was needed to build the railway and road infrastructure before a transport market could take shape.

Therefore a strategy for regional health authorities on regional, national and European levels is needed.

The aim of this strategy is simple.

By creating a common vision of the techniques and services in a comprehensive future RHCN, it will become less risky for European industry to develop and market the required IT services as standard products. But before being willing to invest significantly in this area, industry needs a commitment from healthcare authorities on regional, national and European levels to work in the same direction.

1.7.2   Regional, national and European strategies needed

The most important player in building RHCNs are the local regional health care authorities. These authorities are in most European countries responsible for the co-ordination and continuity of the healthcare services provided in the region. In many European countries they are also directly responsible for delivering significant parts of the services in hospitals and home care units. And as described in section 1.3 "RHCN – state of the art", the political awareness of the need for RHCNs has been growing in the last ten years, and building RHCNs is today a vital part of the regional healthcare policy in many European regions.

To implement the RHCN in the region, the healthcare authority has to set up a regional node and develop a long-term strategy for implementing the different RHCN services in the region.

From the beginning, the regional authority has to establish a Regional Node. To fulfil its function, the node has to provide some basic functionality from the beginning, consisting of an **Internet Portal** describing the services provided, a **key-centre** for encryption (e.g. a trusted third party service), a **Yellow Page** function showing addresses for participating health professionals, and a common **support centre** able to connect and support new users.

The node functionality in the region could be provided by one or more commercial Internet Service Providers contracted by the healthcare authority, and acting as a trusted third-party on behalf of the regional authority. To provide competition between the ISPs, it could be recommended to contract with more than one Internet provider; but a common firewall, common encryption and common support centre has to be established. In that case, it would be possible for each independent user in the region to chose individually from each of the certified ISPs on commercial conditions.

Only a few of the RHCN services could be provided from the beginning. On the contrary, most of the services demand significant organisational changes before being implemented, and other services demands dedicated IT projects. For example, it is normally necessary to reorganise the working process in hospitals before being able to provide tele-medicine expert consultation for health professionals outside the hospital. In the same way, it is necessary to set up dedicated, large scale IT projects involving the local IT providers in the region to make it possible to include Clinical Messaging as a service in the RHCN.

Therefore the regional health authority has to develop a long-term strategy and business plan, showing when and how each of the RHCN services is going to be implemented – starting with the less costly RHCN services like Clinical e-mail, Tele-medicine and Professional Guidelines, and continuing with the more costly and advanced services like Clinical Booking and Clinical Messages.

During the implementation process, the existing organisation and the way of developing cross-sector co-operation in the region need to be changed significantly and fundamentally. For example, before being able to provide Clinical Booking, it is necessary to reorganise the hospitals working processes in order to be able to give immediately the exact time-and-place for a requested investigation. In this way, implementing the RHCN Clinical Booking service could be the enabler to start a BPR process. It could also be an opportunity for the staff and management to reorganise their way of working in a more cost-effective and patient-centred way.

Recommendation for actions at regional level:

- Adopt the vision for building RHCN.

- Make long term regional business plans and project organisation.
- Certificate regional ISPs – and set up a node with basic functionality.
- Implement the RHCN services step by step – and adjust organisation using adequate BPR processes.

Because of the barriers described in section 1.5, the involvement of national healthcare authorities is also very important. Establishing a national strategy, securing national communication standards, and national co-ordination of the regional initiatives, are very important. In some European countries, such as UK and Denmark, official national policies are set up; such policies have significantly facilitated regional improvements. These national programmes are described in section 4.2.

Recommendation for actions at national level:

- Adopt the vision for building RHCN.
- Create national task-force to develop a RHCN strategy.
- Make national security rules and standards for communication.
- Secure co-ordination between regional work and support regional R&D.

Besides the work at regional and national level, European initiatives are needed to create a market for standard products for RHCN services.

European programmes for developing IT for healthcare have mostly been broad frameworks making it possible to develop a wide range of services and products using different technologies. But as described above, the main barrier to developing RHCNs large scale is the lack of standard products; and such standard products are not typically the result of broad defined programmes.

To facilitate the development of a market of standard products, a narrower programme is therefore needed, funding and facilitating the development of RHCN services on a common Internet platform. Such a programme would make it more easy and less risky for European industry to focus their investment on specific, precisely defined services for RHCNs.

Such a dedicated programme could be a natural part of the overall European Information Society Technologies (IST) programme, which in its Vth Framework Programme is aiming along the same lines as described in the strategy building RHCNs.

Together with the development of the regional and national strategies, this could provide a platform for a coherent, firm and co-ordinated strategy ensuring large scale development of RHCNs in Europe.

Recommendations for actions at European level:

- Adopt the vision for building RHCN.
- Develop narrow IST programmes supporting regions implementing the services described.
- Strengthen the European work developing standards for communication.

1.8   RHCNs – the impact and cost-benefits

In the light of the very substantial arguments in favour of RHCNs it is hard to understand why they are not much more widespread in Europe than it is the case today.

If the question was asked to the average health professional or to the average Health Authority manager in the EU "Do you see benefits for the patient in the use of RHCNs?", once the question is clearly understood and the concept of RHCN is explained to them, the answer would almost invariably be "Yes".

Nevertheless, in the EU RHCNs are far from being successful, even now that all the technologies needed to implement them are available off the shelve. Why?

The answer must be found in a dangerous vicious circle where healthcare systems throughout the Union are under strong cost cutting pressure, and there is no spare money to be invested in initiatives with long-term returns. Moreover, healthcare budgets in several countries suffer from a problem of serious rigidity which does not permit savings in one area to be re-allocated to another, different area.

The best strategy to unlock the vicious circle is to provide hard evidence that RHCNs are not only instrumental in improving quality of care, but that they can also release money, which is currently wasted because of poor information and insufficient communication between various levels of care.

Cost savings can be achieved at three different levels:
1. reduction in administrative costs;
2. reduction in duplicated tests, inappropriate or ineffective care caused by lack or loss of information, and unavailability of patients' complete clinical records;
3. improvement of general health, thanks to dissemination of best practice, availability of up-to-date clinical guidelines, thorough and understandable clinical records for all patients, accessible to health professional having the need and the right to know.

The savings released increase by probably one order of magnitude when moving from the administrative savings to the second category of savings, and again by another order of magnitude when going from the latter to the savings due to the improvement of general health.

Unfortunately cost-benefits ratio becomes, in parallel, more difficult to calculate when moving from one level of savings to the next. This is caused by at least three factors:
• the higher number of element intervening in the calculation;
• the subjective nature of some of these elements;
• the time scale in which the savings are released.

The scale of reduction in administrative costs is convincingly demonstrated in the excellent work produced by MedCom of Denmark in association with others[6,7,8]. According to the authors, a non-interactive RHCN based on a mailbox system (store and forward) should get to breakeven after a period of 30 months.

An even more detailed analysis has been carried out by the NHS in the UK. In the context of the Clinical Links project, a cost-benefit analysis has been realised and a Implementation Pack developed, capitalising on the practical experience of the two Trailblazer sites in Avon, and the George Eliot Trust[9].

The Implementation Pack contains both a qualitative and a quantitative analysis of the results, and a series of recommendations for Health Authorities, Trusts and GP practices keen to embark in the implementation of links between Primary and Secondary Care. The paramount added value of the Implementation Pack is the provision of a model, in the form of an easy-to-use spreadsheet, which is meant to be tailored to each individual situation. This enables partners interested in implementing the links to calculate beforehand the cost-benefit they can expect to derive from the network.

The arguments and the criteria developed in Denmark and in the UK can give general guidance to healthcare partners in other countries, but the specific models are not applicable to different realities just as they are.

A major area where care should be taken in drawing conclusions about profitability of a RHCN in other contexts is the level of computerisation among GPs at the inception of the project. In the two countries mentioned above, Denmark and the UK, this level is higher that in most EU countries, especially when compared to the level achieved in the Southern countries of the EU.

If the cost-benefit calculation had to include also the cost of GPs' first computerisation, the conclusions could be rather different; this even without considering the risk and complexity of moving in a single step from paper based clinical records directly to RHCNs.

Separate consideration should be given to those cases where the advantage of telematics is essentially self-evident, e.g. because it reduces the need for expensive or simply impossible transportation of patients. These examples are regions with dispersed populations, such as northern Norway and much of Canada, or remote or inaccessible locations such as islands, oil rigs in the North Sea, etc.

Quite clearly, RHCNs are a non-event if their use in the foreseeable future were limited to communities with special needs, representing a negligible percentage of the EU population.

The authors are convinced that RHCNs will not come about just because they are an effective cost-cutting tool, even if they are also that, but because they contribute vastly to improve the quality of care delivered to EU citizens. Qualitative considerations, particularly related to quality of patient care, are likely to provide a much more compelling argument for RHCNs than a crude financial cost-benefit ratio.

Finally the whole debate about the benefit of RHCNs might turn out to be sterile, just because they will happen by the sheer force of events. Do the hundred of million people who use a PC, a GSM or an office productivity tool such as a word processor ask themselves the question if it is economically justified to buy one of those?

The Health Care sector cannot go against the tide of a world which is more and more interconnected and where physical distances are bridged by communication networks.

The WISE consortium, and the project WISE has brought together, can do their part of the total job by providing more factual elements and more tangible arguments to decision makers who have the power to influence the speed at which RHCNs spread out. These decision makers can decide to invest today in RHCNs rather than tomorrow, and to ride the tide instead of being swamped by it.

CHAPTER 2

2.   RHCNs – MAKING IT HAPPEN

2.1   *Framework Model for a successful RHCN strategy*

The diagram shown in Figure 2 below presents an overview of the various major components that need to be addressed in order to achieve a successful RHCN:

- Environment;
- Organisation, purpose and approach;
- Systems, processes and structure;
- Users;
- Partnerships;
- Resources.

Also shown are the main outputs from a RHCN.

Each major component is made up of a number of areas. These are all discussed in more detail in the sections below.

In developing a strategy for a RHCN, all of these areas should be considered. The strategy should identify where there are issues that must be resolved, and the approach to be taken in meeting the challenge in each area.

First though, we give an overview of the framework model.

2.1.1   Explanation of the Framework Model

Is should be noted that while the Framework can be represented by these dimensions, they are all inter-dependent and impact on each other.

Environment

The development of RHCNs is dependent on the presence and support of a range of environmental factors.

First, it is necessary that **national and regional policy** is supportive and prepared to make **funding** available to create the necessary infrastructure, and to create appropriate **legal frameworks**.

Also all **stakeholders** need to be in support of the RHCN. This includes the information technology **industry** which is prepared to invest in the development of products to support RHCNs. This will be easier if industry is convinced that a **market** exists for these products.

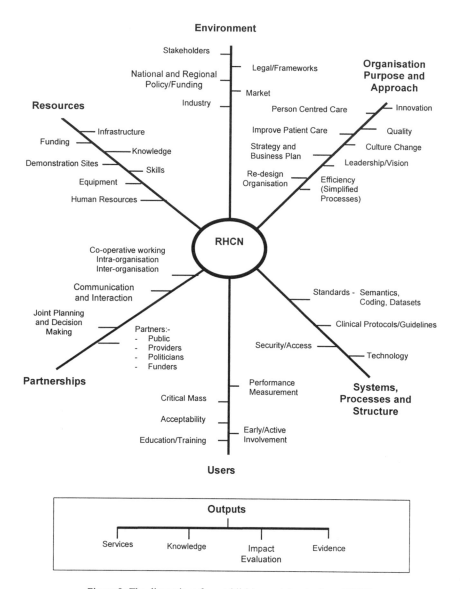

Figure 2: The dimensions for establishing and developing a RHCN

Organisation purpose and approach

The RHCN needs to have an explicit **purpose** and **approach** which member organisations can support.

Central to the value of a RHCN is being able to promote **person centred care**, as it would facilitate better communication and co-ordination between health and social care staff in different organisations.

This should lead to **improved patient care** and also increase **efficiency** since duplication of work could be avoided.

Healthcare organisations across Europe are seeking to continually improve the **quality** of care and performance. The RHCN can contribute by facilitating access to knowledge repositories, and inter-professional communication. Information and data about performance and trends can be more easily configured and extracted and used to plan improvement and **innovation**.

To fully exploit RHCNs and create organisations which use knowledge and new technologies for communication will require **leadership** at all levels of participating organisations and a **culture change** which involves professionals sharing and making explicit their knowledge and decision-making criteria.

Systems, processes and structure

RHCNs will require carefully planned systems, processes and structures, so that resources are fully utilised.

First, **standards for semantics, coding and datasets** (language, terminology and information) will need to be agreed so that information can be transferred effectively between organisations.

Where professional boundary working is to be facilitated, **clinical protocols/guidelines** need to be agreed between the relevant parties.

It will be important to develop **evaluation** and **impact measurement** systems which will be able to demonstrate the gains resulting from the creation and use of RHCN, and to help overcome resistance to change.

The need for new roles, responsibilities and behaviours will be significant, and **human resource** strategies will be needed to help people acquire skills and knowledge they need to exploit the RHCN.

Similarly, as technology enables different ways of doing things, the opportunity for **re-engineering** how resources are configured will present itself. This should be focused on facilitating cross-boundary working and co-operation to improve the quality of experience for the user, and to increase the added value of resource usage at each stage of the process. The goal should be to create **simplified processes**, without unnecessary complexity or bureaucracy.

Issues to do with **security** and **access** will need to be resolved at local, regional and pan-European levels. This may necessitate some legislative changes to create consistency.

The capability of the organisation and the service provided by the RHCN will have to be captured through **performance measurement** systems. These should include financial and linked non-financial indicators.

Users

The staff who will use the RHCN as part of their day-to-day work will need **education and training**. This is to acquire the understanding of the rationale and potential of the RHCN, as well as the practical skills to access the RHCN. The **involvement** of users in the design is important to ensure the **acceptability** of the design of systems and processes, and so that they can see the potential benefits. Incentives and encouragement will be necessary to ensure usage of the RHCN.

Partnerships

In order to make RHCNs a reality, **partnerships** at all levels will have to be created, not least of all to raise funding. These relationships between **planners, providers and politicians** will need to be actively encouraged.

This will enable **joint planning and decision making**. **Co-operative working** will be required at all levels, both **intra-organisation**, and **inter-organisation**. There will have to be ease of **communication and interaction** between all involved to create relationships of trust and goodwill, which will be fundamental to the success of RHCNs.

Resources

The resources required to implement a RHCN include funding to cover the **funding** of **equipment**, the development of new **skills** and the provision of pilots and **demonstration sites**, which will be necessary to persuade and influence users.

Outputs

Finally, what will be the outputs of a RHCN? This is an area which participants in RHCNs should define for themselves. Perhaps the most important output will be the ability to create, share and use **knowledge**, which will **improve patient care** and organisational **efficiency**.

2.1.2   Environment

By definition, environment is a dimension that no healthcare player is able to control. The environment however has an enormous impact on the speed at which RHCNs will develop in the next few years. Hence there is an interest by healthcare players to gain a deep understanding of the environment in which they act, and to devise ways of influencing it.

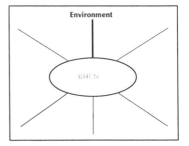

In the following paragraphs the environment of the RHCNs is broken down into these components:

- National and regional policy/funding
- Stakeholders
- Market
- Legal/framework
- Industry

2.1.2.1 National and Regional Policy/Funding

Healthcare in Europe is mainly a non-profit public service that tends to focus on cost containment. Free market principles do not apply to much of European healthcare.

Barriers

- Segmentation of healthcare responsibility: A particular issue for telematic services is that they can rarely be cost justified when looked at from a narrow perspective. Often, the costs and benefits of telematics fall into different organisations, diluting any incentives to invest. A tele-radiology application, for example, which can vastly reduce the cost of radiology consultation for a health area, could have a negative impact on a hospital's accounts. This is because, in most European health services, the hospital has to bear the total cost of investment to implement the service, while the real benefit of such investment is released somewhere else. Segmentation of healthcare responsibility into various levels, and budgetary constraints imposed separately on each of them, can represent a formidable obstacle to the spread of telematic services.

- Culture of public services: Although there is a growing awareness that value-for-money is an important requirement for publicly provided services (and not just for healthcare), the cost-conscious, risk-averse culture of most public services has a number of implications which create difficulties in implementing RHCNs.

- Focus on expenditure: The decisions to invest in IT have been more often based on information on the cost of investment rather than on the assessment of the potential benefits in terms of cost-reduction or improvements in quality or effectiveness. Consequently, the attention of the healthcare managers and the policy makers in Europe has been focused too much on the healthcare expenditure resulting from the introduction of medical and information technologies rather than benefits.

- Investment priorities: A higher priority has been given by the policy makers and managers to investments in new services and medical technologies rather than in IT infrastructures.

- Lack of national healthcare IT implementation strategies: Most European countries lack national healthcare IT implementation strategies, resulting in a lack of structural changes and a lack of direction from government, the professionals or the patients. The stakeholders do not know what they want, except more and better. Even worse, in some European countries, consistent inhibitors still exist in the public administration as regards the utilisation of telematic application in the daily functions of the healthcare system.

- Lack of evaluations of the effectiveness and cost-effectiveness of using IT: Up until now, there have been insufficient opportunities for well-designed evaluations of the effectiveness and cost-effectiveness of using IT for different healthcare activities, hindering consensus building about their value.

Success Factors

- RHCNs, to become a reality, need a federating power, which cuts across the specific goals of individual healthcare players, to promote the general interest of the citizen. Very little can be achieved through local initiatives and trials if the competent National or Regional Authority is not convinced that RHCNs are an indispensable element of future healthcare delivery systems.

Recommendations

- Think global: Because the costs and the benefits of RHCNs often accrue to different parts of the health system, to come about RHCNs require a global strategic vision, which, in some cases, might even require several Ministries to collaborate and share the investment.

- Specific budget for RHCNs: National and Regional policy makers must include in their manifesto the establishment of RHCNs, and put aside a specific budget to implement them.

- Incentives to management teams to spend on linking into RHCNs: While cost containment measures should and will remain in force, the management team of healthcare providers has to be incentivised to spend the money they have been allocated for connecting to RHCNs.

2.1.2.2 Stakeholders

In making the business case for RHCNs, it is important to identify potential key benefits for stakeholders in the community which the network will serve. The many opportunities created by a network are not always visible in the way that applications or products are. We recommend that the matrix in Table 7 below is adapted and applied locally by health organisations to ensure that their own key stakeholders are informed of the potential benefits of RHCN.

Table 7: Matrix of Healthcare Actors and Services

ACTOR / SERVICE	Primary Care Physician	Hospital Clinician	Specialist Clinician	Public Health Clinician	Pharmacist	Nurse and others	Laboratory Technician	Heads of Service	CEO and Senior Managers	Finance / Purchasing Managers	Insurance Executive	Secretary/Administration	Patient
1. Clinical messages	×	×	×		×	×	×	×					
2. Clinical e-mail	×	×	×	×	×	×	×					×	
3. Clinical booking	×	×	×			×	×	×				×	×
4. Shared records	×	×	×		×	×		×				×	
5. Care protocols	×	×	×	×	×	×		×			×		

SERVICE (ACTOR)	Primary Care Physician	Hospital Clinician	Specialist Clinician	Public Health Clinician	Pharmacist	Nurse and others	Laboratory Technician	Heads of Service	CEO and Senior Managers	Finance / Purchasing Managers	Insurance Executive	Secretary/Administration	Patient
6. Mobile & emergency	X	X				X							
7. Home-care monitoring	X	X				X							
8. Tele-medicine	X	X	X										
9. Surveillance information	X	X	X	X				X					
10. Yellow pages	X	X	X	X		X		X	X	X	X	X	X
11. Professional guidelines	X	X	X	X	X	X	X	X			X		
12. Disease quality management	X	X	X	X				X	X	X			
13. Public health information			X					X					
14. Continuing professional development	X	X	X		X	X		X					
15. Reimbursement	X		X					X		X	X	X	
16. Electronic commerce					X	X		X	X	X	X	X	
17. Patient-id	X	X	X			X	X	X	X			X	X
18. Resource management				X				X	X	X	X		

In order for a RHCN to succeed, it needs to provide a return to each and every healthcare stakeholder.

2.1.2.2.1   Citizens/patients

Public opinion has an important role to play in the spread of RHCNs. European citizens are more and more exposed to the Information Society in their daily life (banking, travelling, leisure, etc.); they expect some of these tools to find their way into the healthcare sector.

Healthcare is a sensitive issue at the political level, because everybody has an interest in it. Citizens have a legitimate demand for quality care (as patients) at a reasonable price (as taxpayers). The pressure of public opinion, convinced that Information Society technologies can boost the quality/cost ratio of healthcare, is a formidable force to push politicians to act.

Barriers

- Poor information: Citizens/patients at large are poorly informed about the benefits that RHCNs could bring to them.

- Biased press: The media tend to focus on attention-catching issues such as threats to confidentiality, computer hackers, security of data and often forget to talk about the positive side of RHCNs.

- Fears about the improper use of personal medical data: Personal medical data are a source of information about people's behaviours, potential physical or psychological problems, life expectancy, and hereditary diseases, which are worth money for employers, insurance companies, etc. This generates serious issues regarding the trustworthiness of organisations and individuals having rightful access to personal medical information, and the extent of such organisations and individuals.

Success Factors

- Tangible improvement in quality of care: This can be measured in terms of:
  - sensible application of the latest protocols and guidelines to the prevention and treatment of the pathologies that they are most exposed to or that they have already developed;
  - diagnosis and treatment decided upon on the basis of a comprehensive assessment of their clinical history and their current situation;
  - access to the best specialists around, should the need occur, irrespective of where such specialists are physically located.

Recommendations

- Citizens/patients will have to renounce their right to enforce all the rights they enjoy thanks to European Directives on data protection, and give health professionals having the need to know free access to their clinical records wherever they are.

2.1.2.2.2   Health professionals

Barriers

- Independent attitude of health professionals: Health professionals, as most liberal professionals, have a tradition of working on their own or in small teams located physically in a single place. RHCNs are going to break walls, which have sometimes grown into shields against a competitive pressure considered unethical in medicine.

- Negative side effects: Health professionals will lose comfort, protection and freedom through RHCNs.

Success Factors

The return for health professionals must more than compensate for the loss of so many advantages and privileges. Some of the possible incentives which can be devised for them are:

- Professional enrichment: through exposure to up-to-date clinical information, collaboration with recognised leaders in the medical/scientific sector, personalised continuous training available 24 hours a day.

- Patient management: health professionals will be able to trace a patient, with his/her consent, through his/her evolution inside the healthcare system. A GP will be able to follow his/her patient through the overall diagnostic or therapeutic path related to a problem. A specialist will be able to monitor the convalescence and rehabilitation process of a patient even when he/she has left the walls of the hospital.

Recommendations

- Introduce a financial reward: Several types of financial reward can be devised: bonuses for holding EHCRs, for exchanging clinical data through RHCNs, for booking medical acts for their patients, for participating in GP-specialist networks, etc.

2.1.2.2.3   Health provider management

Barriers

- Conflict of interest: These types of stakeholder are those with the most prominent role to play and, possibly, those with the biggest conflict of interests concerning RHCNs.

  By making information more easily available, the management of secondary care providers enable a shift away from hospital based care towards a community-centred health paradigm. To this extent, they contribute towards undermining their own power; to a lesser extent, the same is true of the management of tertiary care. In addition, this same management is, or will be, asked to invest part of their budget in information services to release benefits which accrue to other healthcare players (Health Authorities, GPs, patients, taxpayers).

Success Factors

- In order to establish RHCNs, secondary and tertiary healthcare providers, as the largest producers of health information, will need to enhance their information systems to handle the clinical information which needs to be communicated and exchanged with the other healthcare providers. Moreover, the information communicated to the world outside must be usable by the recipients, which means that it probably has to be filtered and translated into a terminology which is adjusted to the receiver (GP, community care worker, or even, in some cases, the patient him/herself).

Recommendations

- Strong financial and professional incentives: Strong incentives, both financial and professional, must be given to this category of stakeholder to persuade them to back a process, which, on the surface at least, brings nothing to them.

2.1.2.2.4   Health Authorities

Among all the healthcare stakeholders, Health Authorities are those who should lend to RHCNs their unqualified support, because they have much to gain from the successful implementation in their areas, and very little, if anything, to lose.

Health Authorities of any level should be the strongest force behind the establishment of RHCNs, because the latter help them to achieve most of their institutional objectives.

Barriers

- Awareness: RHCNs are such a clear-cut case for Health Authorities that, if they are not committed to them yet, it is probably because they are not always fully aware of what RHCNs could offer to them.

Success Factors

Health Authorities would expect some of their major concerns to find their natural solution through RHCNs.

- Cost containment, by rationalising the use of resources and by spreading clinical guidelines and protocols, etc.

- More equitable distribution of funding, by furnishing epidemiological data about the population in the catchment areas of health providers, and so enabling a more accurate evaluation of foreseeable healthcare costs.

- More focused health planning, by supplying reliable aggregated information about healthcare consumption, trends, expected demand evolution, etc.

- Better control, by making available on-the-spot comparative information about health providers' behaviour and performance. This, in turn, allows a closer follow-up of unexpected patterns or anomalies in the delivery of care.

Recommendations

- Actively promote RHCNs to Health Authorities: WISE is a step in the right direction to make Health Authorities more aware of the benefits they can derive from the implementation of RHCNs. However, more initiatives of this kind are needed at national and regional level - it is difficult to spread messages through a single event at European level.

2.1.2.3 Market

The vast majority of the money spent in Europe for healthcare is public; similarly most spending decisions are taken by public authorities or publicly controlled agencies. This means that for the RHCN market to mature, Health Authorities and Governments must take the conscious decision to invest money in RHCNs.

Barriers

- Size of the market is uncertain and return on investment is doubtful (how much and when?): In the western world, RHCNs cannot escape the rules of a market economy. The market will not happen at all unless it promises to be big and profitable enough to attract investment from potential solution providers and networks operators.

Success Factors

- With no extra money to invest in healthcare overall, RHCNs must to compete to attract investment, diverting it from other equally important areas. This is affordable only if there is a good assurance of an economic and financial return, and if such return is not too far away.

Recommendations

- Give hard evidence: The WISE Report and other similar initiatives need to address the issue of the return on investment in RHCNs. The more evidence that is gathered to prove that "1 euro invested in RHCNs generates releasable savings in excess of 1 euro over, let's say, 2-3 years", the closer we are to the general advent of RHCNs.

2.1.2.4 Legal/Frameworks

Barriers

- Law and reference frameworks have fallen behind the technological evolution: Law and reference frameworks are slower to evolve than the markets and technologies which fuel them. Today the former have fallen far behind what the market could offer. From the legal and regulatory viewpoint, issues of privacy, security, user authentication, and liability as they apply to RHCNs are not yet resolved. This acts as an inhibiting factor for the widespread adoption and utilisation of telematic services by large user groups. Similarly, the legal status of the electronic healthcare record is still not clear.

- Personal data protection can constitute an inhibitor: The EU directive on the processing of personal data is now to be adopted by member states. It enforces a number of strict rules, which empower the citizen to stop sharing of his/her personal data. This issue may also become an obstacle to the seamless healthcare service.

Success Factors

- Identify all the possible gaps: The good news is that the gaps have been well identified, as a result of the notable contribution of several European projects (mostly but not exclusively from Health Telematics), which have analysed the legal implications of delivering services, and health services in particular, through a network.

Recommendations

- Lend political support to the definition of a legal framework: The legal framework is catching up quickly. Problems such as electronic signature, non-repudiation of messages, and encryption are already being dealt with, or at least debated, in most EU countries.

2.1.2.5 Industry

Barriers

- Fragmentation of the healthcare IT industry: In general, a lack of overall development and investment strategies in healthcare have resulted in a proliferation of local investment decisions, leading to uneven and fragmented development of systems for primary and secondary care, and the growth of a fragmented multi-vendor environment (cottage industry). In other words, there is a tendency that solutions to local needs are developed from scratch, and that these solutions will be created by very small SMEs with little capacity to further exploit and export their solutions.

- Health telematics industry is not there yet: The health telematics industry is not yet a reality today. Several players, most of them small, have just moved the first steps towards building solutions or limited-scale prototypes of RHCNs.

- Pioneers have had their fingers burnt: In general, the large players have snubbed health telematics in general and RHCNs in particular. The disappointing financial results of BT in running NHSnet, and the disaster which RSS promises to be for Cegetel in France, are enough of a warning for other potential providers.

Success Factors

- Ability to build the confidence: This industry, to emerge, needs the guarantee of a market sufficiently large and sufficiently open to induce market players to invest, confident that there will be a good return on their investment. The speed of such return defines the size of companies which can enter this market and stay in it. SMEs, in the European context of overcautious use of funds by venture capitalists (..... is the name actually appropriate for what they do?) can not keep investing for very long before they see a return.

Recommendations

- Communicate investment policy in RHCNs and remain consistent: Big players need to know that money will be spent on RHCNs in a consistent manner for several years, in order for them to invest in RHCNs and RHCN-capable offerings.

2.1.3 Organisation, purpose and approach

In the following paragraphs the organisation, purpose and approach of the RHCNs are broken down into these components:
- Patient centred care
- Efficiency / Quality of care (Improving patient care)
- Strategy & business plans
- Knowledge, information and evidence

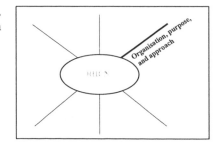

- Organisational redevelopment / culture change
- Leadership/vision
- Innovation

The main goal of healthcare systems is to help the patient attain the best health outcomes in the most satisfying and efficient manner. This implies that health systems should focus on the activities that really accomplish such goals. Very often, however, the role of clinical practice as the main driver of health system policies seems to be forgotten; it is overshadowed by other activities that should only play a secondary role within health systems.

The main objectives of clinical practice are related to the diagnosis, treatment (including preventive measures), and prognosis of the illness, together with a set of activities related to the identification of persons at risk and the prevention of disease. In this context, the organisational culture, its purpose and approach, play a pivotal role in the success of any approach targeting an improvement of the effectiveness of health systems, including the introduction and dissemination of advanced technologies for information processing.

However, networks for healthcare cannot deliver benefits unless the way of delivering care is modified to take advantage of the new possibilities offered by the technology deployed. This will certainly imply that some people will have to modify their working habits, some other will have to change jobs, and in extreme cases some will lose their job altogether. This will inevitably create resistance to the introduction of RHCNs.

Furthermore, there is no point in deploying expensive networks if there is no willingness to re-engineer the processes around such networks. Countries, where health workers have a guaranteed job for life and cannot be re-deployed without their consent (for example Italy), have a definite disadvantage in releasing the benefits of health telematics. They could even be unable to achieve any benefits for a long time because of the inflexibility of their job system. The easiest targets are of course new health institutions, which are created from scratch (for example, the Hospitales Fundaciones in Spain). These can be designed from the very beginning to take advantage of telematics to deliver their services.

Even in the best of the worlds, the introduction of telematics in healthcare will require a massive effort of education, to remove unjustified fears, and to move people away from routines which have changed very little for decades, towards something which is definitely very innovative.

2.1.3.1 Patient centred care

Where patient care has previously been event focused, institutionally based, and specialty driven, a new care paradigm is emerging focusing on a patient oriented approach, aimed at preventing illness, promoting good health and managing chronic illness and long term care. This new paradigm promotes a continuum from home care through primary practice to secondary and tertiary care services, requiring co-ordinated intervention from a large variety of health professionals. RHCNs play a crucial role in enabling this new paradigm to function effectively.

Barriers

- Lack of effective patient education: The patient has too little information on which to base his / her decisions regarding the processes in which he / she is the main interested party.

- Poor integration and communication: There is a lack of integration between primary and secondary/tertiary care together with a lack of communication between the various clinicians concerned with a patient's case.

- Lack of emphasis of health systems on preventive medicine.

- Lack of standards enabling an effective sharing of patients' data.

Success factors

- Systems of population-based risk and disease assessment.

- Increased preventive medicine programmes i.e. systems of disease prevention and health promotion.

- Systems of care based on an effective communication / integration of care providers.

- Effective participation of patients (i.e. patients associations) in the definition of healthcare strategies.

Recommendations

- Healthcare professionals and systems should be able to continuously improve their ability to match services to the needs and expectations of the people they serve.

- Implement a sustained healthcare information infrastructure based on patient care information, which should provide the means to improving the capability to control healthcare costs and enhancing healthcare quality.

- Ensure that appropriate methods and tools enable the patient to be an active, well informed actor in the health system.

- Ensure confidentiality and privacy of patients' data.

2.1.3.2 Efficiency / Quality of care (Improving patient care)

The ultimate goal of the process of care should be to achieve the most favourable outcomes within a defined structure. The new agenda for improving quality in healthcare systems requires the understanding that practice patterns are critical to cost and quality. It also requires the understanding of the meaning of appropriate, efficient and effective care, the role of practice guidelines and protocols as suitable instruments for the dissemination and use of best practice, as well as the need for efficient methods and tools for case management and outcome measurement. Finally, it also requires the understanding of the concepts for continuous quality improvement and the relevance of these concepts to organisational culture change.

Barriers

- Without a clear definition of outcomes it will be impracticable to assess effectiveness.

- The delivery of high-quality patient care is remarkably complex and multidisciplinary, with the processes of care involved in reaching an outcome often differing substantially at the various decision points of the healthcare system.

- Information on what is the optimum process of care regarding most clinical conditions is often lacking.

- Lack of suitable healthcare IT systems.

Most existing healthcare IT systems are focused on administrative data rather than clinical data. Healthcare IT systems are usually poorly designed with poor standardisation and little co-ordination between the different types of healthcare providers (i.e. primary and secondary care), and between these and healthcare authorities. Healthcare IT systems are rarely utilised by clinicians, particularly in hospitals.

Success factors

- A comprehensive framework of automated information, evidence-based medicine, and defined protocols of care, with explicit collection and assessment of outcomes information.

- Use of outcome measurements as the basis for healthcare evaluation and policy making.

- Use of (clinical) quality indicators, as defined by best practice, as the basis for performance indicators for healthcare organisations.

- Increased use of healthcare IT systems by clinicians and patients..

Recommendations

- Promote evidence based medicine / best practice (i.e. systematic reviews, practice guidelines, critical pathways, ...).

- Define the theory and practice of methods to improve clinical decision making to enhance the quality and cost-effectiveness of care.

- Provide detailed information on processes of care.

- Support the participation of patients in healthcare decision making processes.

- Ensure the use of reliable and secure information systems that can support the application of guidelines in the daily clinical practice and integrate them with patient-oriented information systems.

- Promote continuous pursuit of quality as the basis of the organisational culture within healthcare systems.

2.1.3.3 Strategy & business plans

The increasing amount and complexity of medical knowledge, the increasing cost of healthcare services, and the growing demands of healthcare consumers, all contribute to the need for healthcare reform. Healthcare reform is on the agenda in many countries as traditional systems face growing pressures, mostly economic.

Barriers

- Lack of a holistic long term vision of co-ordination, continuity and cross-sector co-operation.
- Current healthcare systems lack coherent models for the management of care provision.
- Lack of consistent regional / national healthcare IT implementation strategies.
- Lack of consistent ethical / legal regulations for the collection and use of outcomes (clinical) data.
- Attitudes of stakeholders.

Physicians and patients, in particular, could be resistant to change because they might fear that 'new' healthcare management models are driven by administrative / economical reasons, thus leading to new restrictions on care provision and loss of clinical freedom. This resistance may however be overcome if both clinicians and patients are the real driving force for future developments in healthcare management (i.e. disease management).

Success Factors

- Increased collaboration of clinicians in the design of appropriate models for the management of healthcare services.
- A robust framework for managing process improvement.
- Consistent plans for handling organisational changes.
- Appropriate educational investments and organisational commitment to learning.
- Appropriate IT infrastructure.

Recommendations

- Set up the information infrastructure necessary for the long term collection and evaluation of outcomes data.
- Regulations for the collection and utilisation of outcomes data.
- The services provided by the system must be highly responsive to the demands of patients and healthcare professionals.
- Processes of care must comply with best practice, and healthcare systems must include sound methods and mechanisms to monitor and assess the outcome of processes of care.
- Healthcare professionals must be empowered in the pursuit of quality, including the means for an optimum communication and collaboration

between healthcare providers, collecting and processing of patient information, and to deliver best practice (i.e. education and training; easy access to data and knowledge, research findings, health outcomes, ...).

- Develop new models for the management of care provision that should be:
  - integrated throughout the healthcare system;
  - capable of handling the overall course of diseases;
  - co-ordinated by means of an effective communication of information between all care providers;
  - evaluated in terms of the effectiveness of all interventions based on collected outcomes;
  - modified via a continuous quality improvement of outcomes.

2.1.3.4 Knowledge, information and evidence

Making decisions well, especially in the clinical setting, is an information-intensive activity in which lack of data about a case can produce considerable biases or errors[10]. Furthermore, clinical decision is a complex task for which many factors might be involved, e.g. education, experience, personnel values, cultural beliefs, social, political, and economical constraints, etc. Hopefully, the role played by scientific evidence in the clinical decision making process is progressively increasing.

Barriers

- Lack of coherent healthcare information systems with appropriate emphasis on clinical data.
- Lack of medical terminology standards.
- Lack of an information / knowledge management culture in healthcare systems.
- Attitudes of stakeholders.

Success Factors

- Large scale population-based clinical trials and epidemiological studies.
- Robust healthcare IT infrastructures.
- Integrated knowledge acquisition and management tools.
- Extensive collection and evaluation of clinical data.

Recommendations

- Ensure there is the information infrastructure necessary for the collection and evaluation of patients' cases.
- Ensure effective sharing of distributed services and related clinical data.
- Promote the use of evidence-based medicine, e.g. by means of computer-based practice guidelines.

2.1.3.5 Organisational redevelopment/culture change

Healthcare organisations / systems are based on complex social, economical and hierarchical interrelationships. The implementation of innovative management models can affect both the human dimension and organisational culture in dramatic ways; these should be kept in mind when introducing new technology (in the broadest sense). Basic principles for a successful culture change include motivation and commitment to excellence of the human system, rather than depending on command and control management procedures. This is particularly true within systems / organisations where most influencing employees are characterised by high levels of autonomy and specialised expertise, such as in the medical sector.

Barriers

- Attitudes of stakeholders.

- Lack of a shared vision committed to the excellence of the human factor in healthcare systems.

- Lack of mechanisms / instruments to assess the organisational performance based on appropriate (i.e. clinical outcomes) quality data.

Success Factors

- Clinical information systems and performance review mechanisms clinically credible and meaningful to clinicians.

- Involvement of clinicians in all aspects of the development and operation of quality assessment / improvement systems.

- Clear definition of educational and behavioural objectives.

- Sustained clinical education programs, co-ordinated by respected clinical leaders, stimulating active clinician participation in educational interactions.

- Individual feedback of clinical performance data, highlighting positive reinforcement of improved practices.

- Incentive strategies to reinforce desired behaviour.

Recommendations

- Promote appropriate training for health professionals.

- Acknowledge good practice and promote its development.

- Develop well designed programmes to improve practice.

2.1.3.6 Leadership / vision

To effect culture change, there needs to be appropriate leadership at all levels of the health organisation / system, in particular for two levels of decision making: managerial and clinical. Firstly, there is a need for an explicit, motivated commitment from health managers to support and promote a quality-based culture. Secondly, it is key to recognise the need for clinicians' leadership in the required change of processes of care, as well as their collaboration in the design of appropriate models for the management of healthcare services.

Barriers

- Lack of a vision promoting a knowledge-based culture in healthcare systems / organisations.

- Attitudes of healthcare managers.

- Lack of comprehensive strategies to change practice and behaviour meaningful to clinicians.

- Lack of incentives to motivate clinical opinion leaders to be involved in the design and implementation of educational interventions.

Success Factors

- Knowledge required of leadership development.

- Interpersonal skills and effectiveness of leaders.

- Clear definition of mission objectives and resources devoted to educational and organisational change programmes.

Recommendations

- Educational efforts should be made to learn and teach the principles of continuous quality improvement and related concepts like outcomes measurement and disease management.

- To promote creative thinking and problem solving throughout the healthcare system.

2.1.3.7 Innovation

The last decades have seen major advances in the understanding of disease and potentially effective treatments, together with an increased utilisation of sophisticated and often expensive technology, and growing costs of medical care. Alongside this unprecedented increase, new treatments are now the expectation of patients, their families, and society in general, leading to an increasing demand for the services provided to the patients.

Barriers

- Lack of effective communication / information infrastructures.

- Lack of consistent regional / national healthcare IT implementation strategies.

- Attitudes of stakeholders, in particular, healthcare managers.

Success Factors

- Organisational commitment to learning and innovation.

- Appropriate re-allocation of resources.

Recommendations

- Implement well designed community / population-based:
  - epidemiological studies to derive relationships between causative factors and patterns of diseases;
  - clinical trials;
  - effectiveness studies;
  - quality of life and functional status assessment studies;
  - healthcare intervention assessment studies;
  - cost-effectiveness and cost-benefit analysis.

- Support standards-setting activities, in particular concerning the development of coding systems and nomenclatures, and electronic messaging for communicating the content of patients records.

- Fund and co-ordinate efforts to develop secure and reliable healthcare information technologies.

- Fund and co-ordinate research efforts to overcome specific IT barriers.

2.1.4   Systems, processes and structure

In the following paragraphs the systems, processes and structure of the RHCNs are broken down into these components:

- Information Models for semantics, coding & datasets
- Clinical protocols and guidelines
- Security & access
- Technology

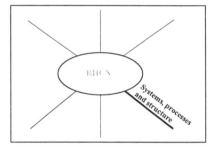

2.1.4.1 Information models & terminology

The RHCN can bring together patient information from different providers to support a shared care model, but differences between providers in semantics and terminology of clinical terms needs to be addressed.

In a RHCN comprising several types of healthcare provider, data is likely to originate from many disparate systems, with variable data quality and a variety of different formats and terminology. To the extent that information in these systems needs to be shared, it is important to reconcile these differences. The intended use of the shared information will determine the degree of standardisation required between data objects; for display-only of patient data sourced from several systems, such information could be displayed as text. In cases where data is used to update other systems or in decision-support applications, common data structures are required, or software to effect the translation from one terminology/coding system to another.

European standards are gradually emerging in health record semantics, terminology and classification (see section 3.3 and Appendix B for further information). For diagnosis, ICD10 is established and already widely used as a classification system. OPCS is also established for operational procedures. For other elements of the health record, there are as yet no European-wide standards, though some classifications are gaining acceptance at a national level. In the UK for example, Read (V3) is promoted as the national standard; in other countries SNOMED is gaining widespread acceptance. As SNOMED and READ are now under single ownership, the convergence of these two systems should provide a firm foundation for a European-wide standard for medical terminology.

The recommendation to RHCN sponsors is to establish working parties across the organisations which will use the network to agree which terminology and coding systems are to be selected and implemented, taking account of European, or at least national, standards where appropriate. The scope of this work should not be over-ambitious in attempting to create a single common terminology for all terms across all providers. It will be more realistic and appropriate to identify those types of information which need to be *shared* and/or *exchanged* between the various parties, and to ensure that there is a common understanding of the meaning and use of the terms - and common data structures - pertaining to that information.

The work required to achieve acceptance of common semantics and terminology across organisations should not be underestimated, even when restricted to information that is shared or exchanged. As health and social care practitioners typically work to different models of care within different cultures, their language and interpretation of terms will diverge as a result. It is vital to introduce any changes to their vocabulary and terms as part of a change programme which makes clear to practitioners the benefits of a shared terminology across providers.

RHCNs can be a catalyst for the re-engineering of healthcare processes, so that these processes are more attuned to a client-centred approach, where clients may have many needs requiring the input of a varied skill-mix of healthcare professionals. Many organisations are now working toward better co-ordination of their staff, either in terms of better communication between independent services, or in terms of team working, where there is closer collaboration in client assessment, care planning and care delivery. The same process of facilitating team working and communication can also be used to encourage the adoption of a common language and terminology.

Barriers

- Incompatible data structures between health providers for many elements of the health record.
- Lack of awareness among users of the need for structured data.
- Lack of agreement on the definition, meaning and use of terms.
- Multiplicity of care models and different functional approaches.

Recommendations and Success Factors

- Adoption of European (or national) classification standards where they exist and can be applied locally by agreement.
- A culture of inter-disciplinary working within the organisation facilitating the development of a common language to describe care practice.

- Implement changes to user terminology carefully as part of a change management programme that includes wide consultation and explanation of the benefits of a shared terminology.

- Consider semantics and terminology issues when implementing a process re-engineering programme – exploit the opportunities for convergence.

- Establish working groups representing the network users to evaluate terminology and coding issues, aiming for convergence of terminology wherever information is shared between different types of user.

- Consideration by the RHCN working groups of the work of CEN/TC 251 (working groups 1 and 2) in defining European standards for data models and terminology (see Appendix B). Develop a strategy and work toward implementing their recommendations over the medium-long term.

2.1.4.2 Clinicals protocols and guidelines

There is growing evidence that rigorously developed guidelines can change clinical practice and improve patient outcome. The current emphasis on evidence-based medical practice is also a driver for the implementation of care protocols and guidelines. However, healthcare professionals are faced with a daunting number of guidelines, which vary widely in quality, and usually contain little guidance in assessing their validity or relevance. This situation could be addressed by developing an electronic searchable database of local and national guidelines which have been critically appraised and abstracted, making this resource widely available on the RHCN, and evaluating its implementation.

Barriers

- Lack of awareness of published guidelines: Healthcare workers and their managers may not be able to invest sufficient time researching the many potential sources of information on clinical protocols and guidelines. Research, collation and validation of guidelines, and their adaptation for local implementation should be separately resourced within the health organisation, then disseminated to healthcare workers through a programme of continuing medical education.

- Concerns among clinicians that protocols may be overly prescriptive: The case-mix of patients can vary considerably from one region to another according to demographic, economic and social factors. Protocols developed on a local basis in one region may require adaptation to implement successfully in another region. Additionally, some of the elements of a care protocol may recommend treatments that cannot be resourced in some regions. If guidelines are implemented without local consultation and adaptation, there is the danger that they will be seen as too prescriptive and inappropriate for the local situation.

- Uncertainty over the validity and authentication of guidelines: Clinical guidelines are now published by many sources and these are often available on the Internet. There are known differences in clinical practice across national frontiers and even regionally. The best approach is for the local clinical community to take on the responsibility of selecting and adapting guidelines for local use, thereby increasing ownership and the likelihood that guidelines will actually be used. For some types of condition, the 'local clinical community' may reside within one organisation, but for many conditions where the patient may receive cross-sector care, the selection and adoption of guidelines should be done as a collaborative exercise between clinical representatives of the agencies involved.

- Uni-disciplinary culture in service planning and delivery: Many health providers organise and manage their services around traditional professional service boundaries. Care is delivered within the capabilities and constraints of those services, in which each profession usually manages its own contribution to care, independently of the other professions involved. Many studies have shown that this service-centred approach may not be in the best interests of the patient, especially for conditions which require the co-ordinated input of a variety of professional staff. Care protocols for such conditions, for example rehabilitation following stroke, and many mental health conditions, will require a co-ordinated approach across professional groups. Organisations which have not begun to work in this way will have difficulty in implementing such a protocol, unless it is accompanied by re-engineering of their working practices into cross-professional team working. Indeed, the adoption of a multi-disciplinary care protocol may act as a driver for this kind of change.

Success Factors

- Executive and senior clinical commitment to the clinical effectiveness agenda.
- Protocols and guidelines maintained on RHCN after consultation and validation, accessible to clinicians over the network.
- Clinicians routinely exchanging best-practice information over the network.
- Use of protocols and guidelines facilitating multi-disciplinary working in the organisation.
- Performance indicators for the organisation include clinical effectiveness targets.

Recommendations

- Assign a Board-level director who takes responsibility for improving clinical effectiveness and ensuring that care protocols and guidelines are successfully implemented.
- Develop a multi-agency strategy for clinical effectiveness, in collaboration with provider organisations sharing the network .
- Appoint a senior clinician to implement the strategy on clinical effectiveness.
- Review working practices, especially of teams, in the light of implementation of care guidelines.
- Publish validated guidelines on the RHCN, and if possible work toward their integration within operational clinical systems.

- Ensure there is a mechanism for feedback on patient outcomes in relation to protocols.

- Implement training on clinical protocols/guidelines as an integral part of the CPD (Continuing Professional Development) programme.

2.1.4.3 Security

Security of information systems is usually defined as data integrity, availability and the prevention of breaches of confidentiality. The confidentiality of personal health information is a vital issue of concern both to the public and health professionals. The European Directive on Data Protection also makes special mention of personal medical data.

The debate on the best approach to health security requirements distils into two main strategies:
1. Investment in a secure private network infrastructure, protected from the internet and other networks by firewalls and associated technology; and/or
2. An encryption infrastructure, overarching the RHCN (or national) domain, but allowing communications to occur over public networks.

Complementary to these strategies, some commentators argue for the adoption of standards enabling the separation of medical data from personal identifiers.

Barriers

- Where the private network strategy has been adopted, rigorous conditions usually apply to organisations and practitioners who wish to become connected ('code of connection' rules). In many cases, significant investment is needed to comply with these conditions, and this has proven to be a limiting factor on user uptake of private networks, especially where they are not centrally funded.

- Competing standards for encryption: this is an area where a European, or at least a national, standard would be of most benefit. Otherwise communications will be hindered by incompatible encryption tools. Public (asymmetric) and private (symmetric) key systems are preferred by different agencies; private key systems incur higher unit costs for maintenance of the keys.

- Where encryption is adopted, key escrow demands by national security services may be unacceptable to some health professionals or their representative bodies.

- Whilst internet/intranet technologies are already becoming established as the global standards for communication, there are currently limitations in SMTP audit trail and security mechanisms, though this area is undergoing rapid development.

- Other messaging protocols which do have advanced audit trail and security mechanisms (e.g. X400) have not achieved widespread acceptance in most European health communities.

- Lack of a nationally agreed protocol in most countries for User Authentication.

- There is as yet no regulatory legal framework in most countries for the rules governing the implementation of networks, regarding: security, data protection, user authentication and the extent and limits of liability applicable to network users.

Success Factors

- Awareness of the emerging national and European guidelines for authorised, recommended security protocols.

- Whether the private network or encryption strategy is adopted (or a combination of these), significant central investment in the infrastructures is required to support them, either by government or by the health insurance organisations.

Recommendations

- Where possible, follow emerging national and European guidelines for security methodology and tools; in the absence of such guidelines, adopt tools which are becoming de-facto standards by virtue of their rapid uptake in the market. Avoid proprietary non-standard technologies and tools which may be technologically advanced, but create a future cul-de-sac for communications with other health organisations that have adopted more standard technologies.

- Encourage the development of a regional health authority policy on medical data security issues; the health authority should then drive the adoption of security standards throughout the health organisations within its region.

- Certification of all networked healthcare practitioners by professional bodies; this would be the criteria for the issue of the appropriate access levels to electronic health records.

- Support the creation of certification organisations to assess and evaluate commercial IT products and systems with respect to their adherence to recommended standards.

2.1.4.4 Technology

RHCNs require a hardware, software and communications infrastructure. A diverse range of technology products are required to support the infrastructure, in addition to the many software applications which will be deployed on the network. In the current environment, there are typically many local area networks (LANs) separately serving individual health provider organisations and hospital departments. Generally, patient-based information resources are compartmentalised within these local area networks; one of the challenges for an RHCN technical strategy is to enable these resources to be shared, as appropriate, throughout the wider healthcare community in the region.

LANs do not become redundant in a RHCN architecture; they will continue to provide services at the local level. The RHCN infrastructure provides the capability to share the information held in these closed local networks with other authorised users in the wider healthcare community. This can be achieved by the implementation throughout the RHCN of EDI, data-warehousing, integration engine and web-enabling software products.

This report has recommended the technologies pertaining to IP (Internet Protocol) as the technology platform for the sharing of information between healthcare agencies, enhanced with encryption technology to prevent unauthorised access to patient information, and EDI (Electronic Data Interchange) products for the exchange of medical record components. For most RHCNs, the technical architecture is likely to be based on that of a commercial Intranet, with an Internet gateway protected by a firewall. The adoption of IP technology means that technological advances in network components and products will be become available to the network provider at a more affordable cost, due to world-wide competition in the market for IP technology.

Bandwidth is a major consideration in the specification of the technology architecture for the RHCN, and in the cost of the service. The bandwidth requirements can be determined from the nature of the applications which will be hosted on the network, together with the number and type of users who will access them. Users needing applications in areas such as high resolution imaging, tele-consultation, tele-conferencing or multimedia education, will need high speed broadband links for those applications. For normal data transfer requirements, such as for most EDI applications, standard Ethernet transmission speeds are usually sufficient. For occasional remote use of the network, dial-up connections over PSTN or ISDN may be sufficient depending on the application. Dial-up connections are likely to become much faster with the expected introduction of ADSL (Asymmetrical Digital Subscriber Line) supporting 2-megabit connections over copper wire.

There is rapid technological innovation in the technologies which support IP connectivity, especially in the area of high-speed broadband networks. ATM, Optical Internetworking, Gigabit Ethernet, packet-switching and innovations in wireless technology are all making possible the availability of much higher transmission speeds on a network backbone. A full appraisal of these technologies is outside the scope of this document, but they are likely to be candidates for consideration in the specification of a high-speed RHCN architecture.

Network infrastructure technologies are an important part of the RHCN, but will probably be managed and maintained by a specialised network service provider. Another level of technology more likely to be supported in-house is the range of systems and applications required to support the integration of data between different systems, and the and sharing of information between different users. Data-warehousing, integration engine, EDI and web-enabling software products are candidate technologies at this level; this is an area where the development of standards is important. and these are now emerging.

Barriers

- Generally, a higher priority has been given by policy makers to investments in new services and medical technologies, rather than to network technology infrastructure.

- There is often a poor understanding amongst policy makers and stakeholders of the potential benefits to be realised by the deployment of telematic healthcare applications in a co-ordinated way across a region. This has resulted in poor investment in the technological infrastructure required to support them.

- In general, the lack of a co-ordinated multi-agency approach to investment in regional healthcare strategies has resulted in a proliferation of local independent investment decisions, leading to the fragmented multi-vendor development of systems for primary and secondary care.

- Most European countries lack national healthcare ICT implementation strategies, resulting in fragmented regional communications architectures with a plethora of incompatible communication protocols.

- The business case for new technology investment is often difficult to prove in an environment where the benefits are shared across different organisations.

- Investment in old legacy network technology has not always demonstrated a clear ROI (Return on Investment); in this environment, there can be a reluctance to invest in new network technology.

- The technologies pertaining to networking are diverse, complex and changing rapidly; decisions to invest and deploy are often inhibited by a lack of understanding of the technology itself within health provider organisations.

Recommendations & success factors

- Ensure that the application requirements, existing and anticipated, drive the selection of technologies adopted for the RHCN; do not deploy advanced technological solutions for their own sake.

- Business cases for technology investment should include not only the revenue implications, but the anticipated qualitative benefits expected from the technology investment for healthcare workers and patients.

- Keep to a minimum the number of suppliers for your network and other technology components; even where standards exist, there is often costly configuration work involved in achieving the interworking of components sourced from different vendors.

- The standard networking technologies deployed world-wide for secure company intranets provide most of the functionality required for a comprehensive RHCN. The early concerns about security with this approach are rapidly being addressed with new solutions by the large commercial interests driving the Internet/intranet development efforts. In the RHCN architecture specification, ensure that scalability is possible, especially in bandwidth, as the number of users and applications increase in the future.

- Choose carefully the ISP (Internet/intranet Service Provider) for the RHCN. The company should be large, have a track record in hosting mission-critical systems with negligible downtime, and have the expertise to deploy the encryption and other security facilities required by patient-based health applications.

- Employ skilled network manager(s) to maintain the RHCN network, *or* outsource the network management and administration to a competent third party with a track record in this field.

- Appraise periodically technology developments, to evaluate the cost/benefit issues in upgrading network components, systems and applications.

2.1.5   Users

Users must play a key role in the development and use of RHCNs. This role may be analysed under the headings:

- Acceptability
- Education/training
- Critical mass
- Involvement

RHCN

Users

2.1.5.1 Acceptability

RHCNs focused entirely on technology will not succeed. No matter how technically elegant or advanced a system may be, it must be acceptable to users for it to be of any benefit.

Barriers

- RHCNs or their components may be difficult to use: RHCNs may be cumbersome, may perform poorly and may be unfriendly. The RHCN must not be an added burden or impose an additional set of tasks.

- RHCNs may not provide benefits to users: Users are busy people; all the time they face demands for greater efficiency and effectiveness. The RHCN must support this and fit in smoothly with routine activities as part of an integrated set of procedures.

Success Factors

- The RHCN must provide tangible benefits to services and patients.

- It must be friendly to use and integrate seamlessly with routine activities of the users.

Recommendations

- Seek to address the working environment needs of the user.

- Strongly support the processes and procedures of users.

- Make the operation of the RHCN user friendly and seamless.

- Seek early gains from the development and involve regional management.

- Make the RHCN reliable and dependable from the user's perspective.

2.1.5.2 Education/training

People must know how to use RHCNs. This requires education, training and a well-established pool of user knowledge.

Barriers

- Poor training of users in IM&T tools: The main focus in training and education of healthcare workers is correctly centred on patient care. There are, however, many facets to this, including the need to avail of modern communications techniques to underpin this care process. This aspect is generally not integrated to any great extent in professional education programmes. The age profiles of user groups may sometimes also have bearing.

- Insufficient time for training: A major difficulty arises in users finding time for training and education, given the persistent ever-increasing demands for services to patients. Resource requirements to accommodate training must also be addressed.

Success Factors

- General IT literacy amongst the users of RHCNs.
- Specific skills in use of RHCN and RHCN services.

Recommendations

- Regard training for the RHCN as an investment that will yield benefits to patients and efficiencies for users.

- Time and resources for training should be provided. Such training must be continuous as the RHCN evolves and develops.

- Training should be included as part of ongoing staff development programmes and should be adapted to suit local needs.

- Train the managers.

- Facilitate extensive communication amongst users on the development of the RHCN.

2.1.5.3 Critical mass

The RHCN cannot exist without a wide range of participants and users. It must be actively and seamlessly used by all to ensure the achievement of its true potential for the benefit of patients.

Barriers

- Poor coverage of RHCN: The greater the coverage of RHCNs the greater the benefits and functionality that will accrue. Successful implementation depends on mutual usage of the various components of the network by many participants. It is difficult to demonstrate wide success with partial coverage.

Success Factors

- The development of a core group of users is essential.
- Peer group enthusiasm for RHCN services.

Recommendations

- Develop pilot components of the RHCN that prove the viability and validity, but be aware that the greater the scope and coverage the more successful the implementation will be.

- Support users in developing various aspects of the network.

2.1.5.4 Involvement

The need to involve the users is a well-accepted fundamental principle in the information systems area, but to get users involved in a fully committed way can be difficult. The RHCN must be 'owned' by its users. It must meet their requirements as extensively as possible. This can only be achieved through active user involvement in the development and running of these networks. This has to be in a very real sense; a token involvement will lead to failure.

Barriers

- Lack of user commitment: The development of the RHCN is hindered when it is not a priority goal for the users themselves, and where there is no serious commitment or ownership among the user base. This can arise through lack of user participation in the RHCN initiative, absence of management support, or too great a focus on the technology as opposed to user needs.

- Pressures on user time: Even if users wish to be involved in RHCN implementation, they may not have the time to provide effective input, due to service pressures, and absence of management support.

Success Factors

- Much success is derived from active involvement of users. This must not only be 'token' or non-participative support.

- It demands serious commitment. This may be organisationally painful but ultimately yields substantial benefits.

Recommendations

- It is a truism in technology developments that users must become involved in developments. This must be emphasised in the case of the RHCN and cannot be understated.

- Involve users at an early stage.

- Ensure project methodologies includes mechanisms and provision for serious user participation.

- Seek real commitment which may at the time be painful for all concerned.

- Support the champions of the RHCN who will make it happen.

2.1.6 Partnerships

In the following paragraphs the partnerships that may be needed for RHCNs are broken down into these components:

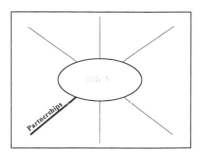

- Joint planning and decision making
- Co-operative working, both intra and inter organisation
- Communication and interaction
- Partners: public, providers, politicians, and funders

No single organisation is able to develop a RHCN alone.

In contrast to "normal" IT systems in healthcare, developing and implementing services and tools for a RHCN needs to be done in co-operation with other, independent organisations. Barriers resulting from lack of cross-sector co-operation have always been a problem in healthcare. But in the area of building RHCNs, these cross-sector barriers are fundamental.

Therefore partnerships and a joint plan have to be built between the different organisations delivering healthcare services to the inhabitants in the region – partnerships involving both private and public providers, and industry.

Barriers

But besides the traditional resistance to cross-sector co-operation, other barriers exist when building RHCNs:

- Before being able to gain any outcome for any of the partners, a significant basic investment has to be made, building the regional nodes and establishing the necessary regional support organisation. No single organisation is interested in making such huge investment alone. This can only be done by establishing cross-sector partnerships.

- The different healthcare organisations in the region have different goals, and are therefore interested in the development of different RHCN services; as an example, GPs are normally very interested in being able to use tele-consultation to access experts in hospitals, but on the other hand hospitals often have little interested in providing such consultation because of lack of resources. Even if different healthcare providers are interested in the same RHCN service, costs and benefits are usually not equally divided between the parties. Normally, for example, the sender of clinical messages has the major investment, while the receiver has the major benefits; however, the opposite is the case for clinical e-mail.

2.1.6.1 Joint planning and decision making structure

The first step is therefore to establish a cross-sector consortium with the task to create and get funding for a joint plan to build a RHCN in the region over some years. To start this process, "someone" has to be the driving force; in most European countries the regional or national healthcare authorities have been shown to take this role. In the Netherlands, Spain, Italy and Denmark, the first actions were taken by regional health organisations starting to build their own RHCNs, and later followed by national programmes to support the regional development. In UK, Norway and France, the start has been made by national authorities followed by regional activities.

In both cases, a national or regional project organisation is necessary together with a joint plan, which identifies which services are needed and the schedule for implementing them. Such a project organisation typically consist of:

- a national or regional steering committee consisting of the main regional health providers, main industry suppliers and involved telecom operators;

- a project manager dealing with the technical set-up of the ISPs, the support organisation and first and foremost the planning and management of the different projects; and

- different project groups dealing with pilot projects – typically one group for each selected RHCN service.

2.1.6.2 Co-operative working

The RHCN is going to support cross-sector co-operative working in the region. From the beginning, therefore, the work to build RHCN services is closely related to the already established work patterns in health, following the formal or informal habits already used in the co-operation between partners. This co-operative work is both inter- and intra-organisational:

- Due to the nature of regional co-operation, the inter-organisational work flows have to be clarified and described in order to develop RHCN services supporting this established work pattern.

- But in many cases also, intra-organisational work patterns have to be adjusted significantly before being able to communicate out of the organisation. If tele-consultation has to be provided from a hospital, administrative and organisational routines have to be established securing access to the experts according to the agreed procedures, while before providing external booking, a hospital has to change its internal work flow, making it possible to book investigations and treatment in the hospital too.

The building of RHCNs therefore often demands restructuring of the existing work flows, both inter- and intra-organisational.

2.1.6.3 Communication and interaction

Building a RHCN involves many different organisations, and effects the work of the employee in many places in the organisation. An effective communication infrastructure, and close interaction between all the project participants is therefore necessary.

But beside this, general information is important too. Both in the pilot phase and especially in the exploitation phase, general information in the form of news letters, PR material, etc., is an important tool facilitating the process. Working across sectors often requires a high degree of political awareness - progress in the projects depends on this awareness.

2.1.6.4 Partners

Managing the whole project needs a regional consortium involving all the main organisations.

But beside this, dedicated partnerships are needed, depending on each of the RHCN services to be implemented in the region.

These partnerships differ for each service due to the fact that each service involves different actors in the region, and different suppliers. In fact, there are four broad groupings/partnerships of the various actors:

- Group 1: Partnerships of healthcare providers, authorities and ISP suppliers: Establishing a regional node needs a deep involvement from healthcare authorities, and from the ISP providers who are going to act as entrusted third parties for the health authorities. But it is also important to involve the users – the healthcare providers – closely from the beginning.

- Group 2: Partnerships of healthcare providers, existing IT system suppliers and standardisation bodies: The RHCN services dealing with structured and integrated communication such as messages, protocols, reimbursement and e-commerce need a strong commitment and involvement of primarily the healthcare professionals, the standardisation bodies and the suppliers of the existing IT systems already in use in the region which are going to develop integrated links to their systems.

- Group 3: Partnerships of professionals and RHCN service suppliers: The services dealing with e-mail, shared records and tele-medicine in many ways develop "stand-alone" systems. They are therefore going to be developed in close co-operation between the users and the industry partners.

- Group 4: Partnerships of public, healthcare professionals, authorities and suppliers: The last group of services are mainly characterised as information systems for a broad group of users, and therefore need the involvement from many sides: public and healthcare professionals representing the user side, authorities representing the official demands and regulations, and finally the suppliers who are going to develop the RHCN services.

The Table 8 below shows the most important partners for each type of RHCN service, and places each service into one of the four partnership groups described above.

Chapter 2

Table 8: Partnerships and services

PARTNERS SERVICES	Public/ Patients	Healthcare providers/ professionals	Politicians / Healthcare Authorities	Existing IT Systems	RHCN Service Suppliers	Standardisation Bodies	Group
The Regional Node		✓	✓		✓		1
1. Clinical messages		✓		✓		✓	2
2. Clinical e-mail		✓			✓		3
3. Clinical booking	✓	✓	✓		✓		4
4. Shared records		✓			✓		3
5. Care protocols		✓		✓		✓	2
6. Mobile & emergency		✓		✓		✓	2
7. Home-care monitoring	✓	✓	✓		✓		4
8. Telemedicine		✓			✓		3
9. Surveillance information		✓	✓		✓		1
10. Yellow pages	✓	✓	✓		✓		4
11. Professional guidelines	✓	✓	✓		✓		4
12. Disease quality management	✓	✓	✓		✓		4
13. Public health information	✓	✓	✓		✓		4
14. Continuing professional development		✓	✓		✓		1
15. Reimbursement		✓		✓		✓	2
16. Electronic commerce		✓		✓		✓	2
17. Patient-id	✓	✓	✓		✓		4
18. Resource management	✓	✓	✓		✓		4

2.1.7   Resources

In the following paragraphs the resources for RHCNs is broken down into its components:

- Infrastructure / equipment;
- Human resources, skills and knowledge;
- Costs.

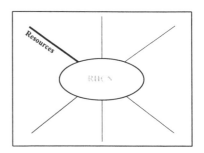

2.1.7.1 Infrastructure / Equipment

RHCNs require at least a basic telematic hardware
and software infrastructure. This basic infrastructure comprises, for example, computers

linked to public networks and local area networks (LANs) with standard peripheral systems (servers, clients, printers, scanners, ...). More sophisticated versions integrate complex information systems such as radiology information systems (RIS), hospital information systems (HIS) and specific devices for radiology and neurology departments (CT, NMR, ...). The RHCN is based, as far as external communication is concerned, on standard and public communication services (e.g. ISDN, Internet protocol suite). Depending on the coverage (number and geographical location of users and systems) and complexity of services and applications (types of information to be exchanged, type of systems, users and on-line services) to be run in the region, the infrastructure components range from very simple "off the shelf" products up to high performance end-user systems and broadband networks.

In addition to the basic infrastructure, specific software components are required which include administrative tools, data bases, solutions to generate multimedia electronic patient records, decision support systems, etc.

Today the market offers most components, and also the support required for the professional services of a RHCN. In addition, there are a growing number of healthcare on-line service providers who can provide a platform for on-line publishing of public healthcare information. Major sources to get a market overview are fairs such as the MEDICA[11] (each Autumn in Düsseldorf, Germany), Healthcare Computing (March, Harrogate, England), or the Cebit (March, Hanover, Germany). Trends in product and service offerings of vendors of IT systems for hospitals are increasingly based on:

- a clear tendency towards integration of information; this is increasingly based on web technologies, which can be considered as the way ahead;
- offering of support for upgrading of legacy systems;
- standardisation, communication and integration as marketing arguments.

In most cases, the potential operators and professional users of a RHCN have technical components and use them on a daily and routine basis, either as stand-alone systems or connected to a LAN. Often, for economic and pragmatic reasons, these components need to be maintained. The barriers with regard to RHCN become apparent if these systems are to be interconnected.

Barriers

The main problems include:

- the potential RHCN comprises a "zoological garden" of hardware and software (different systems, different vendors), so there is a need to integrate heterogeneous systems;
- the need to integrate legacy systems (e.g. proprietary data formats, no support of standard interfaces);
- staff use only basic functions of the up-to-date systems, while the technical features for communication are not considered;
- upgrade of hardware and software is required.

Recommendations

Recommendations and success factors for the planning and implementation of RHCNs are:

- Analyse the available components with regard to their integration capabilities (standard compliance, technical performance), identify the most problematic components, and consider replacing these with state-of-the-art technology.

- Conduct an R&D project with limited coverage and participation, to validate certain components; this must be organised differently in contrast to a real RHCN implementation initiative. The set up of a RHCN for routine use is only sensible on the basis of validated technological components, and requires a detailed work plan that is both comprehensive (covering technical, organisational, logistical, educational aspects) and long term (not only for the implementation phase).

- Specify a scalable and state-of-the-art technical concept for the RHCN. The scalability makes it possible to start with a limited investment, but keeping the option to expand and enhance the RHCN step by step. First hand experiences can be exploited. The figures below show an example of a scalable hardware and software architecture of systems as used by the CHIN project[12] in six European regions. Both clients and servers follow a modular concept covering the hardware and software modules necessary for specific services, e.g. for imaging, communication, security etc. All components follow international standards for communication and formats of medical information as far as possible.

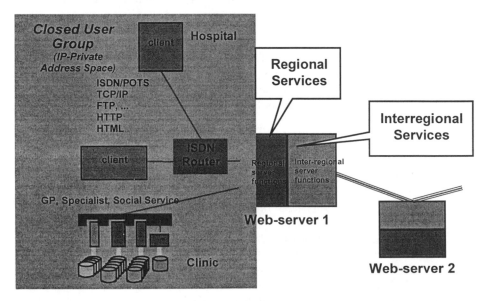

Figure 3: Regional server as central node of an Intranet gateway to public Internet services (CHIN)

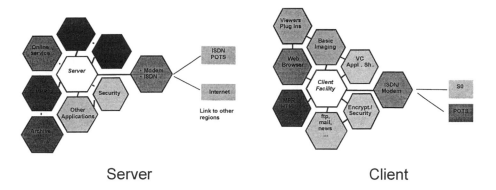

Server   Client

Figure 4: Modular, scalable and standard oriented client/server component concept (CHIN)

- Start the implementation of the RHCN based on existing working scenarios which have the potential to become a success story for the RHCN project. The balance between short term benefits, visibility of results, investments and technical implementation effort should be carefully considered. (Do not start with the most problematic part.)

- Organise permanent technical support for RHCN components.

2.1.7.2 Human recources, skills and knowledge

Essential to the set up of a successful RHCN are the staff, and in particular their motivation to accept a modification to their working processes. RHCNs have to do with new technology; staff who hesitate to use new technology will probably not change. When planning a RHCN, the following arguments and aspects should be taken into consideration.

RHCNs are implemented to help staff do their job better and more easily; it is not an objective to produce additional workload, although during the transition and adaptation period there may be the need to invest more effort. However, it is important that the business and working processes which form the basis for the specific RHCN service allow the staff to understand the benefits of using the new technology. Furthermore, according to the experience of comprehensive RHCN field trials and similar projects, it is a must to include training and education for the users in the RHCN implementation plan, and to identify persons familiar with the technology and working processes as permanent "coaches" and contacts for the users.

The set up and operation of a RHCN requires a specific mix of skills and knowledge. It is necessary to define an interdisciplinary core team comprising IT specialists as well as medical professionals with sufficient know-how and motivation to push the new RHCN based services. This team leads the introduction of the RHCN, it produces specific user manuals, it coaches the operation of the system and manages its further development. There is a need to educate this implementation team, primarily with regard to the needs of users, understanding of their problems, and the way to resolve these problems. The team should be formed with at least a medium term perspective, and not just for the technical implementation work. For smaller units who cannot maintain a core team on a permanent basis, technical and other specialised support needs to be organised using external support.

Recommendations

- Ensure staff understand the benefits of using the new technology.
- Include training and education for the users in the RHCN implementation plan.
- Identify persons familiar with the technology and working processes as permanent "coaches" and contacts for the users.
- Set up a support team, not just for the implementation phase, but also for the medium term.

2.1.7.3 Financial resources

Costs naturally have to be seen in the context of benefits, results, value for money and hence a business case. Clearly, the introduction of new technology and its operation requires investment – investment in hardware and software, in maintenance, in business process reengineering, and in human resources.

Barriers

Often decisions on the implementation of RHCNs depend on pure business considerations. The traditional business case models usual lead to a negative result, in particular in the case of healthcare on-line services for the public. However, the RHCN field trials carried out during the last few years show that the evaluation of financial implications has to be considered not just from a financial perspective.

Recommendations

The qualitative benefits from the perspective of individual user groups, citizens and society as a whole (public health aspects) represent a significant part of the "return on investment" consideration. The emphasis is different depending on the funding arrangements of a national healthcare system, the priorities of the public healthcare bodies and the type of organisation. However, one finding of the implementation and operation of RHCNs in many European countries is that very often it is difficult to prepare a business case for a RHCN as a whole. It is recommended to undertake the value for money consideration for each individual working scenario and for each individual organisational unit separately. On the basis of this analysis, the detailed plan for a RHCN initiative can be optimised. It also becomes clear that not all parts of a RHCN are necessarily expensive. There are scenarios with an obvious and very positive value for money balance; some require only minor investments, while some may require public funding due to a lack of (short-term) business incentives. The return on investment in the case of public access on-line services for healthcare has to be measured:

- by the satisfaction of citizens with and acceptance of a regional healthcare system;
- in public health measured by specific indicators (e.g. health status of the population).

The following examples illustrate these positions:

a) The use of a computer based, networked decision support system for treatment of hypertension with drugs in Norrland (Sweden), based on up-to-date clinical guidelines, led to more adequate treatment and reduced total costs (mainly in drugs) of about 40%. The analysis was based on a test group of 338 patients[13].

b) The evaluation of the routine use of the tele-pathology system in Norrland showed the following results:
   - the time for evaluation was reduced from days to a few hours, which had a significant and positive impact on the treatment strategy;
   - c. 40% of referrals (from remote locations, sometimes hundreds of miles away) could be avoided, leading to considerable savings in transportation costs;
   - improved accuracy of diagnosis;
   - postgraduate education of doctors working in remote places.

c) The comprehensive on-line service for citizens and professionals in Scotland, SHOW[b] covers yellow pages for the Scottish healthcare system, clinical guidelines, and public health information – information provided and maintained by 17 hospitals/trusts, 12 health authorities and 35 other healthcare organisations. SHOW is the leading service in this domain in Scotland (about 90.000 hits per day in December 1998); it has been adopted by the National Health Service in Scotland (NHSiS), and it has become national policy for all NHSiS organisations to develop SHOW compliant sites. However, there was no business case consideration behind the implementation of SHOW – it was driven by public interest an funding; if a business case was undertaken, it is questionable if there was a positive result.

d) In another case in Germany, a trial to turn a heavily used, public and free healthcare on-line service into an at least self-financing service unit failed because people stopped using the service immediately when a monthly fee was introduced. Revenue from adverting alone did not cover the costs, and there were no public means available to rescue the initiative.

2.2   Risk factors and lessons learnt

2.2.1   Risk factors

Experience from current RHCN projects has identified a number of risk areas that can negatively impact implementation of RHCNs:

Discontinuity in management: RHCNs represent a long-term investment: they require long-lasting commitment and perseverance to come to fruition; a "champion" is often the key to success. Changes to key management staff can leave RHCN implementations lacking direction and impetus.

(Macro) Organisational change: (i.e. mergers of health authorities, hospitals etc.) Changes to the organisation of the health system, and to organisations within it, can generate major

b   Scottish Health on the Web, http://pc47.cee.hw.ac.uk/

upheavals. In the worst case, a new change occurs before the previous change had been properly absorbed. This creates risk in a number of ways:

- Changes to organisations are often accompanied by changes to priorities. RHCNs can be one of the casualties.

- Too often, changes to organisations move key people away, leading to discontinuity in management mentioned above. This can happen even when RHCN priority is officially unchanged.

- Changes to organisations frequently result in major demands, in very short time scales, on IT departments; IT managers have been forced to fight a rear guard action, just struggling to keep their information systems afloat. Under these circumstances, work on RHCNs comes a very poor third.

Mismatch of costs and benefits: It is very easy to set up RHCNs so that the costs fall on one party, while the benefits accrue to another. Under these circumstances, the cost-bearing party can be very reluctant to use the RHCN, although there is an undeniable gain to the health system as a whole. This position is greatly exacerbated when multiple services and the infrastructure they are delivered over have different charging processes. Any disincentives on the RHCN arising from these causes can have a direct, immediate and severe impact on the success of RHCNs.

Diverging interests: Interests of individual players do not necessarily converge towards a common goal: e.g. a hospital general manager, who has achieved a high level of efficiency in his hospital, can be rewarded for increasing his hospital output and penalised for promoting de-hospitalisation in his catchment area. This is the opposite of what an effective overall health system may need to aim at.

Lack of consensus between the health professionals and their institutional representatives on one hand, and Health Ministry and health service management on the other hand. Very often there is little selling attempted vis-à-vis the health professionals, to show them the potential benefits of RHCNs. This is exacerbated if there are no services with professional added value planned.

Organisational Culture change: Technological prowess has definitely proven ineffective in promoting the necessary organisational changes and the indispensable change in mindset, which are the fundamental prerequisites for a wide-spread implementation of RHCNs. It has also been found that the genuine and essential enthusiasm of the health telematic community is sometimes slow to spread through the wider user community. Organisational changes (BPR) will arise, and in some settings RHCNs are used as agents of change. This can lead to confusion and serious resistance if not properly handled. Failures are often not because the technical developments fail, rather it is because health authorities and managers underestimate the changes required and the difficulties the organisation will encounter achieving fundamental process change.

Technology led, rather than user led: Projects may become driven more by the technologies rather than the user needs. Health telematics cannot be solely driven by the technology.

<u>Lack of user involvement</u>: Applications concerned with RHCNs demand a high level of direct user involvement. To be successful, they must address the full needs of the users concerned. These needs are not always related to the technology or user interface.

<u>Economic disincentive:</u> The amount of money given to health professionals to equip themselves with the proper systems to generate electronic transactions to replace manual forms often falls far short of covering the real cost. Moreover, in some cases the money is taken from a fund created from forced contributions from the health professionals themselves.

<u>Lack of standards</u>: Agreed standards must be achieved. These standards not only apply to the technology, such as communications and software, but also to areas such as clinical coding, clinical interpretation and common datasets. The lack of standards is a well-known barrier to communicating electronically. Healthcare authorities should play a high profile regulatory role on those issues which would have an impact on the health telematics market. A strong user involvement is also required for application related issues, mainly to identify the requirements and priorities.

<u>Pilots do not always reflect reality</u>: Many applications are developed in experimental/ laboratory type environments without any awareness of the real world where users have to deal with patients, routine distractions and the normal day-to-day activities of providing care.

<u>Pilots cannot achieve critical mass</u>: The size of regional field trials which individual groups have been able to run do not represent a critical mass, able to convince at regional and national level.

<u>Security</u>: RHCNs, in their full implementation, will carry personal medical data, which must be protected. Although there is wide spread agreement on this, at least as far as health professionals are concerned, there is little or no agreement about the most appropriate means to achieve this. Indeed, there is often conflict between health professionals and security services, particularly over encryption. The situation in France over RSS[c] exemplifies this issue. RSS has been widely announced as a secure vehicle for health professionals to exchange sensitive medical data. However, SCSSI[d], an offshoot of the Defence Ministry, have not approved a key long enough to be acceptable to CNIL[e] - CNIL is, by definition, independent from any external influence, and is only concerned about guaranteeing citizens' right to have their personal data properly protected.

<u>Legislative framework</u>: Frequently, legislation does not adequately recognise the issues of transferring information over networks, particularly patient medical data which is especially sensitive. In some countries, legislation prohibits such transfer, unless encrypted.

2.2.2   Lessons learnt

The variety of situations throughout the European Union make it difficult to draw lessons which apply to the whole of the Union. However, the points discussed below certainly have

---

c   Réseau Santé Social, a national network for healthcare and social services
d   Service Central de la Sécurité des Systèmes d'Information
e   Commission Nationale de l'Informatique et des Libertés

general applicability, even though there may be countries where individual points do not apply.

The majority of RHCN projects around Europe have not yet reached the stage of being able to measure quantifiable benefits. However, a general view is that the most significant benefits will be in quality of care, rather than in reducing costs; also that such benefits will be greater if the opportunity is taken to change the organisation and/or organisational processes, to take advantage of the RHCN delivered services.

It is clear that RHCN based services require the co-operation of many different healthcare organisations. This requires significant commitment from within the community of such organisations, and a project "champion"; during implementation, projects are very susceptible to changes affecting the project champion.

Any project aimed at implementing a RHCN is necessarily complex, organisationally if not technically; though interfacing several different systems can be technically complex. This tends to mean that such projects have a long life cycle, during which technology can change, local priorities can change, or national health service circumstances can change. All these can affect the project, sometimes positively, but more often negatively. There is therefore a strong benefit to be derived from gaining early "wins" for the project participants.

The effort required to achieve a common understanding of data semantics is often significant. It is very easy to underestimate the effort needed to achieve this. Early pilots can help with this.

The complexity of RHCN projects is significantly affected by the (non-)availability of standards, particularly application related standards - these are the ones that most affect linking the various end-user systems that RHCN applications often need for maximum benefit.

For developments to be successful they must:
- reflect the business and technical strategies of the organisations concerned;
- become integrated parts of these technologies;
- work towards supporting the routine business processes of the organisations concerned.

The context in which a system has been implemented can have significant impact on how it will be used. The environment in which the user operates can determine how efficient any system becomes.

Significant training is usually required and new skills may have to be developed.

Security deserves a special mention as a potentially formidable obstacle to the implementation of RHCN. The situation today in the various trials around the EU varies from total neglect of the problem to paranoia about possible confidentiality breaches. Neither of the two extremes is acceptable, and the current situation of disparity between one country and another are a clear symptom of lack of consensus and immaturity around this issue. Even within the same country, different schools of thought promote different solutions for data protection and security. Uncertainty in such a critical aspect, particularly important for medical data communication, could paralyse the implementation of new RHCN and bring to a stop the existing ones.

RHCNs need to be based on a win-win pattern. RHCNs can not be implemented against the will of the healthcare professionals.

Power struggles and unrest in the healthcare sector can only be exacerbated by an attempt to implement RHCN.

Divergent interests and internal struggles among different parts of government can destroy the credibility of RHCNs and fuel scepticism among target users. Government should do all the necessary housecleaning before RHCN are publicly announced, and implementation activities start.

Change needs to be sold to users. Health professionals, as with any other segment of the population, are suspicious of change and reluctant to embark on it. Prepare all the arguments to sell the benefits of RHCNs, and to appease the fears they can raise among users.

2.2.3 Do's and don'ts for implementing RHCNs

Summarised below are the main do's and don'ts, drawn from a representative sample of RHCN protagonists from around Europe. These are tactical issues, which need to be considered within the framework of the strategic recommendations set out in section 1.7.2 above. They are structured according to the main headings of the Framework set out in section 2.1 above.

Environment
- Explore other ways of funding RHCNs e.g. pharmaceutical industry (need to deal with issues of probity and control).

Organisational Purpose and Approach
- Adopt a step-wise approach, rather than a global approach trying to do everything for everyone all at once.
- Know where you need to make changes to the organisation.
- The organisation needs a very clear business strategy, which includes the IT strategy and shows that the RHCN represents the option that will give the required benefits.
- Need ability and strategy to manage change. May need to step backwards before moving forward.
- Need to consider who owns the overall process of care.
- Try to get decisions taken nationally.

Systems, Processes and Structure
- Rely on the market for *de-facto* standard technology solutions; do not adopt obscure or experimental technical options.
- Ensure adequate technical evaluation of infrastructure and applications, especially with regard to interoperability.
- Ensure technical solution(s) adopted allow scalability as requirements evolve.
- Differentiate clearly between evaluation tasks and implementation tasks.

- Adopt standards where they exist, with the agreement of all key stakeholders.
- Find ways of delivering early benefits to users, however small.
- Promote a culture of inter-disciplinary team working wherever appropriate.
- Develop a multi-agency strategy for clinical effectiveness, with clear lines of responsibility for implementation.
- Use the network to publish best practice guidelines and to encourage their use.
- Recognise the importance of, and get support for, a multi-agency policy on data confidentiality, supported by data security applications on the network.
- Make use of work published by other RHCN implementations - avoid re-inventing the wheel.

Users

- Focus on user requirements.
- Stick to reality of users.
- Make sure users have benefits from use.
- Diagnose the resistance to change – need a profile of users. Need to know who will support the change.
- Educate users early so they can take good decisions.

Partnerships

- Understand networks first, which means developing confidence and creating horizontal organisational structures rather than hierarchical ones.
- Need communications strategy to ensure that everyone knows what is going on. All actors need to feel that there is transparent leadership.
- Dilemma of issue of procurement and the need for partnership for development – find ways to work in partnership with a company.
- Create partnership between providers/suppliers.

Resources

- Establish clear funding policies.
- Recognise that significant effort will be needed from all participants.
- Identify training requirements.
- Create tight project/resource plan.
- Adopt very strict implementation phase.

Outputs

- Need to be able to demonstrate to people the consequences and the why.
- Define scope of project very clearly and the phases. Need to have clear understanding of this by staff.
- Use RHCNs to integrate legacy systems and to add value to existing investments.
- Demonstrate impact and gain.
- Conserve organisational energy.

CHAPTER 3

3. RHCNs – THE FUTURE (1998 – 2002)

Taking as a starting point the vision for a RHCN set out above, this section looks at the barriers to realising the vision, the products and services needed to deliver the vision, and the market for such products and services, to which suppliers will need to respond. It concludes with a summary of expected RHCN developments in a number of countries within the European Union.

3.1 Products and services needed, 1998 - 2002

There is still a long way to go before RHCNs are really established in Europe. The technical issues of linking systems with one another are not now the main issues. Rather, the principle issues are:
- the gaps to be found in the functionality of the end systems that RHCNs could help to connect; and
- organisational barriers, which are extremely difficult to overcome.

Nevertheless, the medical community and the IT industry will move ahead. The products and services needed are directly derived from deficiencies and barriers described in section 2.1 above:

- Integrated and easy to use practice administration, patient data management and communication systems, with seamless integration of communication functions.

- Local support for RHCN infrastructure. Most providers of IT systems today only provide support either for the LAN or for the WAN / intranet services.

- Compatible and common security solutions, e.g. medical professional ID-card with standardised private keys, trust centres.

- Attractive service packages of public and professional RHCN services.

Europe is far from being a homogeneous market in several fields, and healthcare is certainly an area where there is no clear sign of convergence towards a single model for healthcare delivery.

In determining the products and services needed for RHCNs as envisaged in this section, it is useful to distinguish between the different information flows which potentially constitute the traffic carried by a would-be RHCN:
- administrative transactions;
- booking service;
- clinical information;
- clinical protocols and guidelines;
- multimedia information.

These are discussed below.

3.1.1   Administrative transactions

In numerous countries (for example, Denmark, France or the UK), there are several administrative messages, which could with advantage be exchanged through RHCNs instead of on paper. They cover several different aspects such as:

- patient registration (in those countries, e.g. Italy or the UK, where citizens are registered with a specific GP);

- items of service (in those countries where doctors and health institutions are paid on the medical acts performed).

These services are the easy target for starting RHCNs: both Healthlink and NHSnet in the UK, and RSS in France, three of the largest healthcare networks designed up to now in Europe, have been initially developed to carry this type of data.

Administrative data are easy to handle (IT was invented a few decades ago to handle administrative data after all) because they tend to be structured, codified and therefore unambiguous.

Moreover, if there is an area where health authorities have a strong negotiating power, it is where the information exchange is required to provide administrative data for payment or reimbursement purposes.

In addition, confidentiality issues are less relevant, although not completely absent, when the personal information provided about a patient does not include any clinical data.

Finally, when a decision is taken about exchanging administrative data in electronic format, the obligation to do so for health professionals and health institutions tends to be strong. For end user system suppliers, this represents enough of a guarantee that their investment will produce a good return, if they enhance their products to exchange such messages, because of the wider market they will be able to supply products to.

Stimuli to health professionals to acquire a compliant product vary from a straightforward allowance to buy it (the Netherlands, Denmark where specific incentives are paid to healthcare professionals for using electronic health care records or EDIFACT messages), to a charge for any manual (rather than electronic) transaction they generate from a certain date onwards (France).

The evident conclusion is that RHCNs are likely to start from handling administrative data and will evolve at a later stage to handle other types of data.

This conclusion should not create disappointment in the reader, because this first step is already able to provide a huge amount of statistical information that would remain otherwise beyond reach. The simple possibility of linking a medical act to a health professional and to a patient could tell a lot about healthcare delivery in a geographical area, if such information can be rightfully exploited, while protecting the privacy of citizens.

3.1.2   Booking service

In several health systems, there is a clear imbalance between offer and demand of some medical services. Over time, this has built up waiting lists for these medical services, together with poor interaction between healthcare providers and patients waiting for the given service. As a result, an appointment, when it is finally scheduled, might turn out to be inconvenient for the patient, or even the notification of the appointment to the patient might just go astray. This generates in turn a number of appointments where the patient does not attend, with a waste of capacity for the healthcare system as a whole.

Interactive booking could go a long way towards resolving this problem, because the patient is enabled to negotiate the date and time of an appointment and because he/she gets confirmation on the spot.

The benefit of an on-line booking service grows with the opening of the healthcare market and with the increase of the number of healthcare suppliers entitled to offer medical services to a given patient in competition with one another. This opening up is a normal trend even in healthcare systems where there used to be a rigid patient-GP-secondary care provider association.

RHCNs are ideally suited to offer an on-line booking service, but there are several obstacles to overcome. These range from the inadequacy of the secondary care provider appointment system, which is frequently still paper based, to a strong opposition by heads of service to open their diaries for booking by others.

The latter attitude is frequently justified by logical arguments, such as the impossibility to code all the complex rules associated with booking of a certain medical act (prerequisites, facilities, personnel, etc.), or the need for a head of service to assess personally the priority of a series of requests. Sometimes, however, the real reasons for such an attitude have to be sought in a protective posture against intrusions from outside in the running of a secondary care department. This posture might be considered outdated in a world where the new mottoes are "integration among different levels of care", "continuity of care", "disease management", etc., but it remains difficult to eradicate.

3.1.3   Clinical information

The transmission of clinical information and its subsequent integration into clinical records at different levels of care is where RHCNs could release all their potential benefit. Unfortunately it is by no means the easiest area to address.

Problems lie at different levels:

- Inadequacy of current Electronic Healthcare Clinical Record (EHCR) systems.

  For the exchange of clinical data not to remain a mere replacement of paper by an electronic hard copy of a paper document, such data needs to be structured and codified according to coding systems understood unambiguously by both sender and receiver.

This is unfortunately far from being the norm. The penetration of EHCRs in Europe is still low and it is not true that all EHCR systems currently installed are oriented towards the codification of the medical information (symptoms, diagnosis, treatment, etc.).

- Classification and codification criteria.

Even when this is the case, there is little guarantee that two health professionals would codify the same symptoms in the same way. Evidence of this problem is the fact that in large secondary care institutions, the codification of the medical information for producing Minimum Data Sets, DRGs or other similar summaries, is carried out by specific staff, especially trained to do so.

The consequence of the above is that full transparency of medical information is a couple of generations ahead of us, even provided there is a clear decision to include classification and codification as a subject of study for the medical doctors of tomorrow.

- Personal data protection laws.

A further obstacle to the wide dissemination of services for the exchange of clinical information might come from a restrictive interpretation of the European Directive on the protection of personal data[f] and of its transposition into national laws. There are examples (e.g. CNIL in France) of such demanding restrictions imposed on the exchange of personal medical data and of such strict rules to verify the consent of the patient, as to render the exchange of clinical data through RHCNs almost impossible, or at least not viable from an economic point of view.

Despite the problems discussed above, within the 1998-2002 horizon some basic services can be expected to be included in the offering of RHCNs. In order of likely availability they are:

Laboratory Test Result Return: This is the number one service in terms of actual implementation. This is because the output of practically 100% of laboratories in Europe is already in digital format, and because there are widely accepted standards (including EDIFACT in some countries such as Denmark, France and the UK) for the exchange of structured messages. Moreover, laboratory test results represent the biggest volume of data that health professionals handle in their daily practice.

Hospital Discharge Summary: Most hospitals in Europe are already bound today to produce a summary with information about the hospital stay of the patient; this is often in electronic format. Depending on the standards in use in the various countries the summary can be more or less rich in clinical information but it always contains some, which can be easily retrieved and integrated in an ECR system.

Diagnostic Procedure/Outpatient Consultation Result Return: Any medical act, which is carried out by a technical department within a secondary care provider, generates a

---

f   Directive on the Protection of Individuals with Regard to the Processing of Personal Data and on the Free Movement of such Data. Directive 95/46/EC.

report, which today is mostly in free text. With limited effort, it would be possible to codify some of the fields and so to improve the usability of the information contained in the report.

Drug Prescription and Dispensing: It is a relatively easy service to tackle because of the high level of computerisation of pharmacies throughout Europe. The solution through RHCNs, with a central storage of prescriptions, should be assessed against the use of cards as information carriers, in regions where health cards are in distribution.

3.1.4 Protocols and guidelines

RHCNs are an ideal vehicle to disseminate clinical protocols and guidelines. The level of sophistication in the implementation of the protocols and guidelines can vary from the simple dissemination of multimedia documents and abstracts, to the development of real workflow applications accessing shared EHCRs and supporting shared care protocols involving healthcare professionals and paramedical staff scattered over a geographical area.

Within the 1998-2002 time horizon, applications in support of shared care protocols are likely to be included in the offering of RHCNs. Such applications, although rather advanced in terms of features, address a networked way of working which has become already rather popular among health professionals for the treatment of some major and/or chronic diseases.

3.1.5 Multimedia information

While some services might need multimedia information exchange (e.g. second opinion between specialists, tele-consulting, distance learning) this remains a niche requirement for the near future. This is somewhat surprising when considering that the main emphasis of Health Telematics in the IV Framework Programme was actually multimedia. One might argue that the Programme was in advance in comparison with the market, which is still far from having solved the problem of exchanging alphanumeric data on a regional, national or trans-national scale.

3.2 Industry and market trends - European and global

3.2.1 Evolution of demand

The likely evolution of demand for services is a direct consequence of the major trends in healthcare, which are broadly the same in all the developed countries.

De-hospitalisation: the patient should be kept in hospital the minimum time required to treat acute episodes. Services in support of de-hospitalisation can be categorised as follows:
- sharing of patient's clinical and nursing records;
- clinical messaging (structured and coded);
- dissemination of clinical protocols and flow control;
- tele-consulting and tele-monitoring.

Delivery of health care at the place of living: the health system should be designed to deliver, whenever possible, care where people live instead of taking them from their normal setting. Services in support of distributed delivery can be categorised as follows:
- sharing of patients' clinical and nursing records;
- tele-monitoring and alarms;
- tele-consulting;
- self-compiled feedback reports.

Continuity of care. Various health professionals and paramedical staffs acting around a same patient should be aware of each other's interventions and should follow a clinical path, which is known and shared by everybody. Continuity of care requires to cut across several level of care managed independently from one another. Services in support of distributed delivery can be categorised as follows:
- sharing of patients clinical and nursing records;
- tele-consulting;
- dissemination of clinical protocols and flow control.

Patients co-management of their health: patients should become not only clients of the health system, but they should also co-manage their health in collaboration with health professionals and health authorities. Services in support of patients' participation in their health improvement/maintenance can be categorised as follows:
- access to a subset of individual clinical records through intuitive human interface;
- distance education on health issues;
- prevention campaign dissemination;
- tele-consulting.

3.2.2   Products

All the application services mentioned in section 3.2.1 can be provided with today's technology, without any need for further technology oriented R&D.

In some cases, existing products/prototypes might need further engineering and packaging to become more robust and easier to install. Mass production of health specific information tools (e.g. EHCR, clinical protocol modelling) will push their price down, and will render the cost of implementing health networks more affordable.

The biggest savings in terms of implementation costs, however, can be achieved through a clear commitment to introduce precisely identified and unambiguous standards at European and national level, and by a widespread adoption of them by software suppliers. This applies to both messaging (e.g. EDIFACT, HL7, ICD 9/10) and program-to-program communications for interactive applications (e.g. standard APIs).

Once again the same conclusion can be drawn: for the large-scale penetration of RHCNs throughout the European Union, the standards that products use to communicate with the rest of the world are much more important than their internal architecture.

3.2.3 Market

3.2.3.1 Value

No reliable data exist today to estimate the value of the market for RHCNs and health telematic services in general.

An estimate of the value can however be obtained by combining together a number of elements, which are easily quantifiable.

Let us start from the cost element. Educated guesses are possible as to the cost of providing such services: they are derived from the Study into Telemedicine Using Euro-ISDN[14]. According to the results of the study, and with a small additional elaboration of data, the cost of providing an average basket of RCHN services to a region with a population of some 5.000.000 inhabitants should be in the order of 10-15 million Euros a year. This equates to a cost of less than 3 Euros per person and per year. For arguments sake, double this cost to 6 Euros, to allow for all possible underestimation.

Price on the other hand is related principally to the perceived value for the buyer. The perceived value is strictly related to the economic and financial benefit that the user derives from the service. Clearly, this has to be greater than the cost of providing the service for a supplier to enter the market.

Following this reasoning, price per person per year could be positioned in the 6 to 12 Euros range; this remains far short of 1% of the average healthcare expenditure per person per year[g]. Nobody could ever doubt that better integration among different levels of care, and better patient information management, that RHCNs make possible, is not going to save at least 1% from the total EU expenditure.

Following the reasoning above, the total potential market value is comprised between 2,25 and 4,5 billion Euros a year for the whole of the EU.

Fragmentation of the market is another factor which is going to influence the attitude of potential suppliers towards entering it.

The number of individual networks in the union can be estimated by adding up the number of independent health authorities, which have the size and the spending power to build a RHCN for the area they are responsible for. Precise data for Denmark, Italy and the UK, where there are respectively 15, 21 and 124 such authorities, have been, extrapolated to the whole of the European Union. A reasonable estimate is that the total number of potential buyers for RHCN in the EU ranges between 400 and 500, with each individual network covering, on average, a population of 500.000 to 1.000.000.

Dividing the annual value of the market by the number of independent buyers, an average value per contract of between 4,5 and 9,0 million Euro per year can be obtained; this is an value which should appeal to larger players and not just to SMEs.

---

g   Roughly 1386 euros per year according to table in section 4.2.2

3.2.3.2 Segments

No major evolutions are expected in terms of market segmentation. Various categories of networks can be identified depending on their purpose. Of course, the same network can belong to more than one segment if it combines several types of services.

Metropolitan/Regional Booking Networks

This type of networks responds to the logic that citizens resident in a given metropolitan or regional area should be allowed to select the medical service they need from all the potential providers established in the area, both public and private. This implies that citizens should be given a dynamic picture of the healthcare offering, including information about waiting time and price.

Metropolitan/Regional Booking Networks have a market in those countries where a few factors are present:

- Demand for healthcare services exceeds offer of such services, at least for some specialities, creating waiting lists and the need to book medical services.

- Health professionals and/or patients have freedom of choice about where to get medical services.

- There is a cultural or political environment favourable to open up the secondary care appointment list to enable authorised people from outside to book into them.

Messaging networks

They offer the secure exchange of personal medical data through messaging. Messaging will be preferably structured, coded and based on international standards.

They are the bread and butter of all healthcare networks, because their interest is undeniable independently from the specific organisation of healthcare in a given region.

Integrated Regional Networks

Networks of this kind foresee the integration of health information throughout an entire region. A single health professional or health provider will hold Electronic Patient Records for their patients. These will then be aggregated up, into regional databases that contain global data for epidemiological, health planning and budgetary control.

To achieve their full span, Integrated Regional Networks need a structured and hierarchical healthcare organisation, where the healthcare planning and control function is clearly identified.

Tele-consulting networks

Tele-consulting networks are built fundamentally for selling expertise outside the normal catchment area of a hospital, at a very competitive cost.

To sell expertise successfully in competition against more conveniently located secondary care providers, a tele-consulting provider must offer a clearly perceived benefit. For this reason, this type of network can only be mounted by tertiary care providers, or by hospitals with well-recognised centres of excellence "sellable" outside regional boundaries.

Scientific/epidemiological networks

Networks of health professionals, mainly GPs, who feed a central database with very detailed, but anonymous information about their patients. The central database can be later exploited by authorised users for different types of analyses.

Strictly speaking, these networks do not need to be regional, because what they attempt to provide is not a comprehensive representation of health in a specific region, but rather consistent data coming from samples of population belonging to different geographical areas for comparative analysis.

Shared care networks

They are specialised networks aimed at improving continuity of care for patients suffering of chronic and/or serious diseases. The services offered are centred around protocol and clinical guideline dissemination, and shared Electronic Patient Records.

Even if there are no intrinsic reasons for keeping the geographical span of such networks small, known initiatives in this area tend to be very local in scope. This can be perhaps explained by the need for a close collaboration between various levels of care; this is easier to reach among people who know each other personally.

Inter-sector networks

Looking beyond the purely health related network, there is a need for networks linking relevant information across sectors; for example, for young people, there is a need to share information with education and juvenile justice systems.

However, resolving the issues to bring about networks for health will absorb most of the effort available for the moment. Inter-sector networking is likely to take a while longer.

3.2.3.3 Applications

End user applications are key to the large-scale deployment of RHCNs in the European Union.

The market offers today commercial applications which can already, or could easily, provide all that is needed to implement RHCNs.

The situation is however unsatisfactory in several respects:

- Market penetration: EHCR, which are a fundamental requirement to take full advantage of most telematic services for healthcare, are not sufficiently widespread among health professionals and healthcare providers in several European countries.

- Openness: Even if modern applications have been designed to exchange data with the world outside, most of the application currently installed in healthcare are closed and self-contained, remnants of a time when blurring of borders between different levels of care or different players within a level was not the dominant trend. Legacy applications are not, generally speaking, good at sending, receiving and integrating data coming from external sources.

- Standards: Despite the courageous effort by the European standardisation bodies to elaborate standards for healthcare IT, these standards are far from being adopted by member countries and by application suppliers. Applications adopting standard communication protocols and formats are an essential prerequisite to fuel RHCN deployment.

3.2.4   Comparison between EU and the rest of the world

The European Union is not, in general, the ideal setting for RHCN. The density of population in the Union is high, mobility of patients and health professionals is facilitated by an excellent network of transport, and clinical skills are abundant. Nevertheless, the European Union is far from lagging behind the rest of the world in terms of technology and expertise for RHCN.

This is the result of a number of factors:

- Areas with sparse population (Northern regions of Sweden) or with major transport problems (mountains and islands, oil rigs in the North Sea) do exist in the Union, and they are often combined with a particularly harsh climate.

- Urban areas are often so congested that travelling time, even over rather short distances, can take a long (and often unpredictable) time.

- The average patient has a high level of education and shows a sophisticated demand for healthcare services, which is not always satisfied by local offerings.

- The pace of life is so fast, especially for some segments of the population (e.g. managers, entrepreneurs, top professionals) that convenience and speed of access to healthcare delivery is regarded as a very high priority.

- Ubiquitous access (anywhere, at any time) is considered more and more an indispensable feature of any class of services including health services.

- Public funding for RHCN and health telematics in general has been provided by the European and national authorities for a number of years. Though small in absolute terms and, regrettably, spread over a large number of projects, such funding has planted the seeds for a full-scale implementation of network services.

All in all, Europe has more to teach than to learn from the rest of the world about RHCNs. Such a theoretical leadership, however, has not resulted in sizeable business for the European industry yet, probably because the market for RHCNs is far from being a reality yet.

3.3 The need for standards

This section describes the need for standards, looking at the background, the problems, and the goals. For additional information, Appendix B Healthcare Standardisation Organisations describes the current position on the organisations involved in setting standards in healthcare.

3.3.1 The scenario

The organisation and delivery of healthcare services is an information-intensive effort. It is generally accepted that the efficacy of healthcare operations is greatly affected by the extent of automation of information management functions.

Traditionally, the healthcare environment has always been very "alert" and sensitive to technological progress, and has benefited systematically from the results of R&D. The evolution of clinical tools is an example of the permeability and fast integration of technology in health systems.

But, when referring to Information Technology, the situation changes dramatically. A simple observation of the market of products shows how few are the solutions on offer for the healthcare environment, whether off-the-shelf, or plug-and-play. Conversely, most of the applications running in this sector show a high degree of proprietary solutions, isolated, producing as an outcome real "islands" of IT products.

The dichotomy that can be detected between users and technology, that lack of adaptation to a new culture, is a factor to take into account when implementing EDI and, in general, telematics. This fact may help to explain the difficulties of progressing from pilot to full scale implementation, or the solutions that are apparently available and easy to implement, but which fail, to our puzzlement.

In the past two decades, healthcare institutions, and hospitals in particular, have begun to automate aspects of their information management. Initially, such efforts have been geared towards reducing paper processing, improving cash flow, and improving management decision making. In later years, a distinct focus on streamlining and improving clinical and ancillary services has evolved, including bedside (in hospitals and other inpatient environments) and "patient-side" systems (in ambulatory settings).

Within the last few years, interest has developed in integrating all information related to the delivery of healthcare to a patient over his or her lifetime (i.e. an electronic medical record). It has also been envisioned that all or part of this electronic medical record should be able to be communicated electronically anywhere as needed.

It is common today for the average hospital to have installed computer systems for: admission, discharge, and transfer; clinical laboratories; radiology; billing and accounts receivable; to cite but a few. Often these applications have been developed by different vendors or in-house groups, with each product having highly specific information formats.

As hospitals have gradually expanded information management operations, a concomitant need to share critical data among the systems has emerged. Comprehensive systems that aim at performing most, if not all, healthcare information management are in production. These systems may be designed using a centralised or a distributed architecture.

Network technology has emerged as a viable and cost-effective approach to the integration of functionally and technically diverse computer applications in healthcare environments. However, these applications have developed due to market structure rather than through a logical systems approach; they are therefore often ad-hoc and idiosyncratic.

In summary, it is important that both vendors and users are not faced with the problem of supporting incompatible transaction/communications structures. Instead, a framework must be developed for minimising incompatibility and maximising the exchange of information between systems.

3.3.2   The problems

Healthcare application standards today come from the main centres of development in Europe and the United States. Australia, New Zealand, Canada and Japan are also participating in the process. Currently there is a lack of co-ordination between national development organisations, which adds to the confusion. On the positive side, communication between the two largest centres of development, the United States and Europe, is improving rapidly.

Electronic data interchange (EDI) has been in use for many years. The first users implemented local solutions that typically allowed one party to communicate with one or more other parties using a proprietary message and perhaps also a proprietary communications protocol.

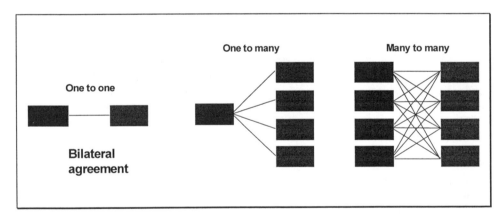

Figure 5: Non standardised communication

In order to support many-to-many communication there is a need to establish common communications procedures. Such common procedures have to be defined for all of the communication levels involved. From the messaging point of view the most important are:
- definitions of information concepts and the coding of these concepts;
- definitions of the information elements to be exchanged and the structure between these information elements;
- definition of a syntax specific message;

- definition of communication protocols.

Each of these levels is standardised by one or more specific standardisation organisations. Examples of these standards are EDIFACT and X.400.

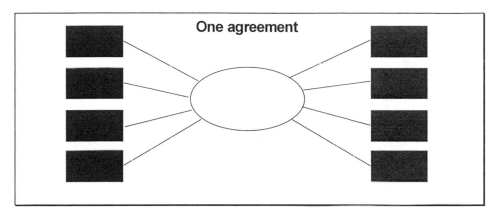

Figure 6: Standardised communication

3.3.3 The goals

With the development of policies that aimed to reduce the barriers to trade within the European Union, standardisation was no longer seen as an obstacle but as an encouraging element facilitating the construction of the single market. As the market was to consolidate, the European standards would substitute the national standards, helping to reinforce it.

That was in the early 80's. During 1985, a first decision to use European standards to support the adoption of European directives (that should harmonise the national regulation for health and safety) implied the movement of expertise from national to European work. This movement led to the work programme for developing more than 10.000 standards (through the European standardisation bodies CEN, CENELEC and ETSI).

In 1991, a Cupertino agreement was signed between CEN and ISO (International Standardisation Organisation) to facilitate the alignment of European and global standards. That important decision implied a European yet a global feature of the work. As a result of this policy, in 1996 more than 40% of the European standards had their corresponding identical ISO standard.

It is known that although healthcare is one of the largest sectors in society, the relative weakness of standards has been one limiting factor for the optimal use of information technology. One of the positive aspects of the internationalisation is the availability of standards already used in various organisations that could serve as input for the international work.

It is also clear that, when talking about healthcare telematics, there are a number of inter-sectorial standards that should be considered as a prerequisite in order to guarantee the interoperability between systems in different healthcare organisations.

One of the main problems that healthcare standards have to face, not only at international but also at the European level, is the fact that many different systems and different concepts and terms are used to describe healthcare facts and telematics.

3.4   *Security - problems and solutions*

This section does not attempt to provide a full discussion and explanation of all the issues affecting security. Rather, it provides an overview of the security issues affecting services provided over Regional Health Care Networks.

Broadly, there are three types of security threats that can affect services provided over RHCNs:

1. Ensuring data in a message is not corrupted; for example, test results must not have critical values changed.
2. Ensuring false massages are not sent; for example, if best practice protocols are available from a Web site, then a medical practitioner wishing to rely on such a protocol needs to know it has been set up by a reputable person/body.
3. Protection of content against eavesdropping - a particularly sensitive issue with personal medical data, which has specific safeguards in the European Directive on Data Protection.

While all these problems could be alleviated if not solved by associated manual processes, in practice dependable computer-based solutions are needed for ease of use and acceptability of the systems.

Possible solutions are either to protect the network against third party intrusion, which would protect against all three threats above, or to use encryption techniques.

Encryption techniques can be used to protect against the threats identified above in the following ways:

•   For threat 1 above, add a digital signature using a cryptographic system, or encrypt the data; this can be done using either a public key (asymmetric) system, or a private key (symmetric) system.
•   For threat 2 above, add a digital signature using a cryptographic system, or encrypt the data; this can be done using either a public key system, or a private key system.
•   For threat 3 above, encrypt the data; this can be done using either a public key system, or a private key system. An alternative which may be acceptable is to separate each transaction into two messages: one containing the medical data, the other the personal identification; the two parts of the transaction are then "married" using a unique "key".

Protecting the network against third party intrusion implies a private network, with secure gateways at every point where there is a connection between the private network and any public network. This requires a significant investment in network infrastructure. In a large network with diverse organisations, it is also difficult to guarantee 100% compliance with the processes and procedures needed to secure the network.

Using a cryptographic system also requires a significant investment, this time in key management. Given the number of actors even within a region, using a symmetric key system imposes an impossible burden on key management. Systems being trialled therefore use a public key system; under some schemes, this is used to encrypt a "session" key for use in a symmetric key encryption algorithm for performance reasons. Using a cryptographic system gives greater flexibility as to the network used to deliver the service - even internet could be used.

There are a number of projects funded by European Commission to trial security schemes using trusted third party key repositories to hold and authenticate public keys for use in asymmetric cryptographic systems.

Affecting the use of any cryptographic system is the attitude of national security services. Security services view the general availability of strong (i.e. very secure) cryptographic systems as posing threats to law and order, should criminal or hostile persons gain access to them. Security services therefore often require key escrow facilities to be built into trusted third party key repositories. This is often unacceptable to the medical professions.

CHAPTER 4

4.   RHCNs – A PERSPECTIVE BY COUNTRY

This section describes the present situation in each country, covering:
- organisation of healthcare provision;
- information flows;
- use of IT in healthcare;
- current status of RHCNs, regional or national programmes, etc.;
- the "state of the art" in industry products, services and plans for RHCNs;
- known plans, trends and likely future development in the next few years.

The section is restricted to core components relevant for a RHCN. The necessary peripheral systems (e.g. HIS, PACS or patient management and administrative systems) are only covered with respect to the interfaces required to integrate these systems into RHCNs.

Before looking at each country individually, an overview of the European and global situation is presented, followed by a number of general points.

4.1   European and global situation in RHCN

Regional Health Care Networks (RHCNs) are being developed in many countries around the world. This applies both to the traditional state-based health systems such as those generally found in European countries and to the more independent structures similar to those that exist in the United States. Both customer (patient) expectations, and the emergence of alliances and links between different providers, demand integrated networks to enable the sharing of patient data. Pressures exist globally to improve efficiency and reduce costs. Quality and continuity of care is also a common theme. Healthcare organisations are looking to exploit their RHCNs to help them meet their objectives on these fronts.

One of the key goals of all health services is to provide a continuum of care for patients. There is much emphasis on delivering that care to patients in the setting that is most appropriate to their needs. This can be in a primary, secondary or community (home) environment. Patients themselves, however, rightly expect their contacts with healthcare to be seamless. In this seamless environment, they also demand that the flow and availability of the information about them matches their service needs.   All this requires a strengthening of linkages between services, including the sharing of patient information between the care agencies involved, and the breaking down of organisational, regional, national and international boundaries based on the use of a variety of new technologies.

Current medical and diagnostic devices enable specialist treatments to be provided away from the traditional clinical environment.   This is driving changes in the way communication takes place between different providers. This not only requires a regional network infrastructure, but also agreement on standards, security and confidentiality requirements, together with facilities for co-operative working that allow the optimum use of scarce health sector resources across organisational boundaries.

There are many examples of initiatives around the world, which have developed and demonstrated the sharing of healthcare information between different healthcare providers.

These use a variety of advanced technologies to meet the needs of patients and their care providers.

A number of factors are contributing to growth in this area, including the development of encryption techniques, the wide investment in global high speed networks, and the prevalence of the Internet throughout the world. It is, however, necessary to look beyond traditional telematic confines. Technologies such as digital radio networks, mobile telephony, digital TV, cable networks and interactive telephone systems are also presenting new opportunities.

While RHCNs present opportunities to improve the treatment of individual patients, they also allow the streamlining and simplification of many complex processes. They help to dilute real or perceived organisational boundaries.

Most of the issues that arise are not technology related. The move to RHCNs is a complex process that is influenced by many factors including technical features, human elements, organisational inertia and business processes. Tele-medicine demands a wide range of standards for it to operate effectively. These are not all technical. There are professional concerns and issues on information content. Many legal issues need to be addressed and resolved. Europe has taken the lead on many of these, and moves are being made to advance such developments on a global basis. In industrial sectors, acceptable standards exist in many spheres of activity. The same progress needs to be achieved for the RHCN.

RHCNs have enabled tele-medicine to cover a wide variety of applications. The scope for further expansion is vast. It is already widely used for remote consultation, diagnostics and surgery. The 'virtual hospital' is becoming a reality. Interactive health education helps the switch from reactive to proactive intervention and illness prevention. The use of electronic commerce is moving beyond the limits of the commercial environment to areas such as health and social services.

RHCNs are becoming an endemic component of health services. Service providers would find it difficult to deliver care without them, and any future initiatives will be based on the 'taken for granted' availability of such networks.

4.2   National developments in RHCN, 1994 - 98

4.2.1   Healthcare organisation

It is clear from the discussions below that there are two principle dimensions to the provision of healthcare delivery within Europe:

- Organisation: a state run national (or regional) health service v. a "liberal" service provided by independent health professionals / organisations;

    In the extreme case of a national health service, all hospitals are state run, GPs, physicians and specialists etc. are salaried employees of the state, either directly or through hospitals etc. Patients will tend to be "registered" with one GP, who acts as gatekeeper to the rest of the healthcare system.

    In the extreme case of a liberal system, hospitals are privately owned and operated, and health professionals are paid for activities undertaken, patients treated etc. Patients have the right to go to any healthcare professional they wish, and seek second, third and fourth opinions.

- Financing: funding through taxes or national insurance (social security) payroll deductions v. (private) insurance / payment by users.

In practice, health systems tend to be a mix of these variables. In the diagram below (Figure 7) each country is positioned in a matrix of these two dimensions. The majority of countries have publicly funded healthcare, whether through taxes or national insurance contributions, while provision tends to be publicly controlled, although in several countries GPs are self-employed. In most countries, there is also an element of privately funded healthcare.

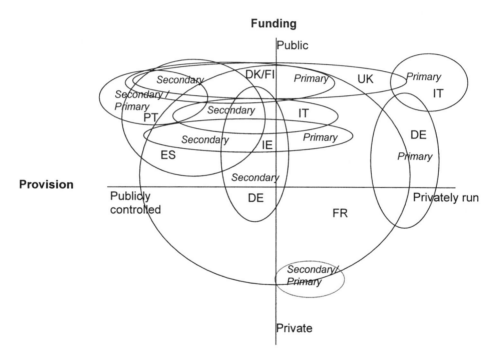

Figure 7: European healthcare organisation

Both these dimensions have an impact on the introduction of RHCNs:

- In a "liberal" system it is more difficult to establish the community of interest that is needed before a RHCN can be established, whereas national health services tend to be able to establish a central agenda for the introduction of RHCNs.

- Even in a national health service, the funding and benefits of RHCNs often accrue to different budget centres; this makes approval and funding of RHCNs difficult. This situation is greatly exacerbated in a liberal system, where individual health professionals have to pay for services directly.

4.2.2 Healthcare expenditure

Table 9 below provides comparative figures on healthcare expenditure as a % of GDP, both total and funded out of public expenditure, for the countries of the EU. It also shows the change in expenditure over the last ten years. Actual expenditure per head of population (PHoP) over the ten years has risen significantly, in line with the increasing prosperity of EU countries.

Table 9: Comparative Healthcare Expenditure[h]

	1996	1986	1996	1986	1996	1986
	Total expenditure as % of GDP		Public expenditure as % of GDP		Total expenditure per capita in euros PHoP	
758	8.0	6.9	5.7	5.3	1497	885
Belgium	7.8	7.4	6.8	5.9	1463	800
Denmark	7.6	7.9	6.2	7.0	1953	928
Finland	7.4	7.4	5.8	5.9	1182	776
France	9.8	8.5	7.3	6.5	1715	972
Germany	10.5	9.2	8.2	7.1	1951	869
Greece	6.8	4.4	5.2	3.6	761	281
Ireland	7.0	7.7	5.2	5.8	1093	505
Italy	7.8	7.0	5.5	5.3	1357	741
Luxembourg	6.8	6.0	6.2	5.3	1832	816
Netherlands	8.6	8.0	6.2	5.8	1513	845
Norway	7.9	7.2	6.5	6.3	1651	895
Portugal	8.3	6.9	4.9	3.7	917	385
Spain	7.4	5.6	5.8	4.5	955	405
Sweden	8.6	8.7	7.2	7.9	1435	1018
UK	6.9	5.9	5.8	5.0	1128	616

Notwithstanding the increases in healthcare expenditure shown above, or perhaps because of them, there is a growing pressure to ensure value for money in the use of healthcare resources. Along with developments such as clinical audit, healthcare authorities are looking for quality improvements through better use of information, and sharing of information, about a patient, to ensure the optimum outcome for any treatment.

4.2.3 Information flows

In order to use information better, and share it, the information needs to be exchanged between the various healthcare actors.

These information flows are both clinical and administrative. While the latter tend to be specific to each country, clinical information flows are essentially similar.

---

h   OECD - www.oecd.org/els/health/fad_1.htm- (Oct 1998)

Figure 8 shows these main clinical flows; while there are minor variations from country to country, these are not significant for the purposes of this report. In the context of Figure 8:

- 'Diagnostic Services' refer to services which require the presence of the patient, such as radiology, MRI, etc.;
- 'Specialists' can include dentists, opticians etc., where appropriate to the context of the healthcare organisation;
- 'Home Care' can include such services as physiotherapy, midwifery, etc., where appropriate to the context of the healthcare organisation;
- 'Hospital' includes tertiary as well as secondary care hospitals.

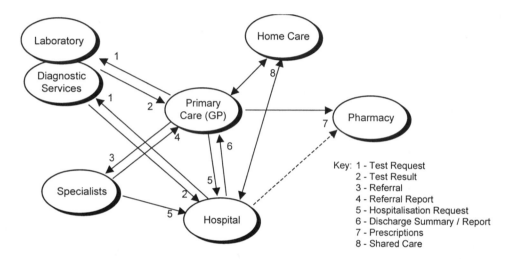

Figure 8: Clinical information flows

It should be noted when considering the above flows that in some countries, the "logical" units are part of the same organisational structure; for example, laboratories are often part of a hospital.

4.2.4   Service offerings

It is helpful when considering RHCN products and solutions to divide them into two major groups:

1. Complete products and service offerings. These are based on a dedicated network infrastructure, with security components which meet the legal requirements for the communication of patient identifiable data. They support end-systems for users, and operate on-line services with content relevant to RHCN subscribers. Typically, they will provide services which directly support the clinical treatment of patients.

2. Content only on-line service (information) providers. These are typically operators of public or password protected Web servers with content relevant to specific user groups, structured more or less appropriately to the users' needs; they can be international, national, regional or even local in scope. While this type of regional healthcare content/service is not of itself a RHCN, it represents

an essential asset for a RHCN. However, if it is not integrated into a RHCN of the first group, it can only cover public information, and is therefore less useful for professionals with regard to their daily working processes. There is a huge amount of information published this way.

In the sections below, attention is focused on the first group; however, some major providers of "content-only" services are also identified.

4.2.5 Penetration of EHCRs

In Figure 9, the penetration of EHCRs within primary care within UK and The Netherlands is shown; these are the two countries for which there are good records.

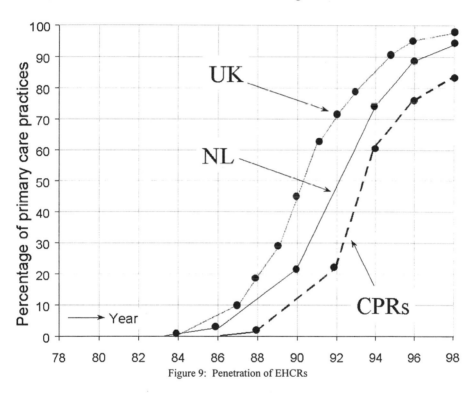

Figure 9: Penetration of EHCRs

4.3 Denmark

4.3.1 Healthcare organisation

Denmark has a public healthcare system; this is paid for by taxes, and managed by the Danish counties. The counties own almost all hospitals, and the county pays for most secondary care services delivered by private GPs and private specialist doctors. Home care is also mainly publicly funded, and is owned and managed by the 284 local authorities. GPs use laboratories and other investigation services based in and paid by the hospitals.

Approximately 85% of healthcare is financed via taxes. Primary care doctors are private, but mainly controlled (regulated) by the authorities. 15% is paid by individuals – either directly or via private insurance. Most of this is drug costs, but there are also a few private hospitals (also publicly regulated).

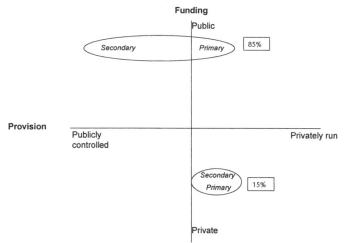

Figure 10: Funding and provision of Danish healthcare

There are 15 counties in Denmark, covering from 200 - 500.000 inhabitants. Most counties have four to six local hospitals and one or two larger hospitals; these range from small local hospitals with 100 beds to large university hospitals with more than 1.000 beds.

Since 1990 legislation has ensured free choice of hospitals between counties, and inside each county. The free choice is made by the GP, who acts as a gatekeeper for the entire healthcare sector.

4.3.2 Information flows

Almost all communication in healthcare in Denmark is regional: between the hospitals in the region, and between hospitals and GPs in the region. Only a minor part crosses regional borders between local hospitals and national university hospitals, and almost no communication crosses national borders.

Most of the communication is textual, covering the classical information flows such as prescriptions, laboratory results and so on. This communication is normally done by ordinary mail, or by local parcel services set up in larger cities gathering laboratory requests or prescriptions. There is little communication of images and pictures. Consultation with experts is normally not formally organised, but ad hoc phone calls from GPs to hospitals are used instead.

About four million letters a year are communicated between the partners in healthcare in a typical region, and 40 million for Denmark as a whole.

It is not only on paper that Denmark has a single-stringed health system with the GP as gate-keeper to the other treatment services. This position as a nodal point means that the GP receives far more cross-sector information than the other parties in the healthcare sector, both in absolute and relative terms. However, this communication is very simple:

the majority of the communication to and from general practitioners can be described in just six communication flows:

1. national health insurance accounts;
2. prescriptions;
3. laboratory results and requests;
4. referrals and discharge;
5. X-ray requests and results;
6. communication with home care.

4.3.3 IT systems in healthcare

The development of hospital information systems in Denmark started twenty years ago; today all hospitals use patient administration systems, and all laboratories have computerised laboratory systems. For the moment, systems are being implemented rapidly in the radiology area, and a national programme for introducing Electronic Health Care Records (EHCR) in hospitals was launched by the Ministry of Health in 1996.

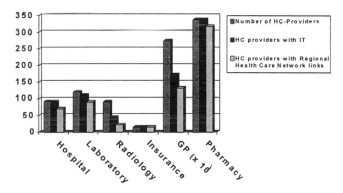

Figure 11: IT in Danish healthcare

During 1995 to 1996 almost all GPs (80%) have implemented EHCR systems, and all pharmacies have used IT systems for the last five years. The use of home-care systems is very limited today.

IT Providers

About 30 different IT providers offer IT solutions to Danish healthcare; half of them offering solutions to secondary healthcare, half of them to primary healthcare.

Almost all IT systems used in healthcare are developed in Denmark and delivered by Danish companies. In the hospital area, the market is dominated by one large IT company, Kommunedata. This is a publicly owned company, founded at the beginning of the seventies by counties and local authorities. 11 counties are primarily using Kommunedata in the hospital area and four counties are using other Danish IT providers.

There are 12 IT providers to GPs; three of these cover 70% - 80% of the market.

The market for pharmacy systems is covered by four IT providers; one of these is owned by the pharmacy organisation. Only in the laboratory area are "foreign" IT providers used.

4.3.4 Current status of RHCN

The developments in healthcare since the seventies have resulted in introducing new, specialised parties in health. Twenty years ago, the patient was a patient at his family doctor or at the local hospital, and almost all diseases were cured by one of these parties alone.

In Denmark, as in all other European countries, this is no longer the case. New specialised functions have emerged like the home care area, the specialised laboratories, the physiotherapists, more expert hospitals, and expert clinics. No general medical department exists any longer in any Danish hospital, and the GP acts more as gatekeeper to the entire healthcare system than as the isolated family doctor. The result of this development is of course a growing communication between the different, co-operating parties in health; this is distributed by normal mail, by the use of phone, and by local transport services set up between the doctors, hospitals, pharmacies and laboratories in the region.

In the late eighties, interest in electronic communication between the various parties in healthcare increased. On the initiative of the Danish Association of County Councils, therefore, local projects introducing electronic communication between hospitals were started in Vejle and Silkeborg, amongst other places. The projects were financed by the large, public owned IT-company Kommunedata. Together with the report "IT across (Sector) Boundaries" prepared by Danish Hospital Institute, these activities helped to draw attention to the need for cross-sector communication on the political level.

In parallel with these projects, a prescription experiment involving pharmacies and GPs was carried out in Copenhagen in 1990. This experiment was groundbreaking for building RHCNs in Denmark, and since that time almost all RHCN projects in the healthcare sector have built on this technological basis:
- standardisation of the information content making it possible to communicate from all to all;
- EDIFACT syntax;
- use of existing telephone lines for communication;
- use of VANS (Valued Added Network Services) suppliers and traditional e-mail based mail-box technology.

Due to the huge political interest in improving co-operation between the different parties in healthcare, three large projects started building RHCNs in three different regions in Denmark:
- FynCom – the Funen County Network;
- Odder – the Århus County Network;
- KPLL – the network for laboratory communication in Copenhagen.

All three projects take the technology used in the first Copenhagen project as their starting point.

In order to prevent each Danish region reinventing the wheel, the Funen County Council in 1992 submitted a proposal for organising a joint nation-wide project to which all parties should contribute: MedCom, the Danish Health Care Data Network. Two years later, MedCom was started with the goal of building a national standardised communication infrastructure in Danish healthcare, connecting all different parties (GPs, hospitals, pharmacies etc.) and building up RHCNs in each of the Danish counties. MedCom was funded one third by the Ministry of Health, one third by the counties and one third by healthcare professional organisations and industry. The total budget was 2 million euros.

In the period 1994 to 1996, standards for the most frequent information flows in regional health were developed and verified in 25 regional pilot projects spread all over Denmark. Each of them developed and verified the use of standardised communication for each of the classical data flows; all of them involved virtually all hospital IT systems, and the majority of doctors' EHCR systems used in Danish health.

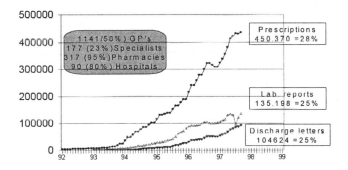

Figure 12: Number of messages and number of participants in September 1997

Since 1992, the communication and the number of participants in Danish RHCNs has grown. Today more than one third of all prescriptions, discharge letters and laboratory results are exchanged electronically between hospitals, laboratories, GPs and pharmacies, and more than 1.000 GP practices, 200 specialists, 300 pharmacies and almost all hospitals are connected to the network.

The technology structure differs from county to county, taking as the starting point the IT structure already in place in the region. In the Funen County, the hospital and laboratories are connected using in-house formats and a central mainframe system as a node, while the GPs and pharmacies are connected to a national VANS operator (DanNet) using normal telephone or ISDN lines.

Due to the huge focus in Denmark on the classical flows, the development of other parts of the RHCN have been slow, except for building high-speed imaging networks:
- in Viborg County, X-ray images are exchanged through a local ATM network between the hospitals;
- in the Copenhagen area, a large scale wide area picture network has been built up;

- in Funen, Nordjylland, Vejle and Frederiksborg counties, general information systems for general practitioners are used.

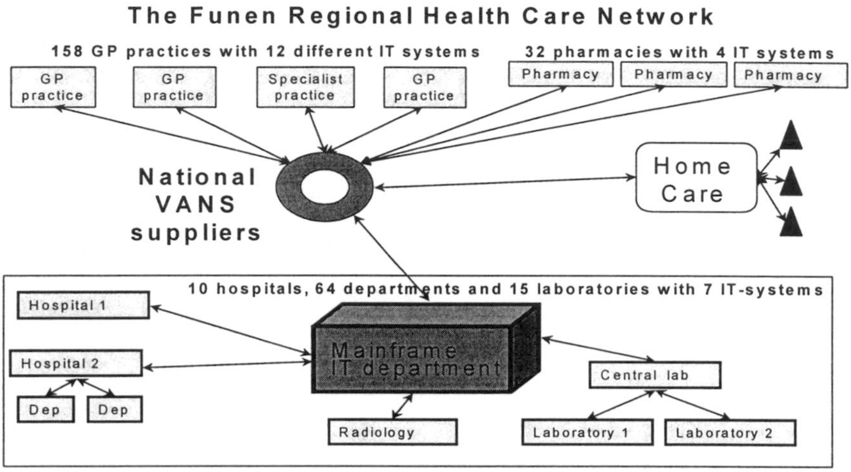

The Funen Regional Health Care Network

158 GP practices with 12 different IT systems   32 pharmacies with 4 IT systems

Figure 13: The Funen Regional Health Care Network

4.3.5   Industry - companies, products and services for RHCN

The RHCNs in Denmark have so far been focusing on EDI standardised integration between existing IT systems; almost all IT systems have in-built solutions for the classical information flows in healthcare. Two VANs suppliers (Kommunedata and DanNet) are the only suppliers providing mail services to general practitioners, pharmacies and hospitals.

4.3.6   Future development of RHCN, 1998 - 2002

4.3.6.1 Trends and future development

The focus in building RHCNs in Denmark in the years to come will be the MedCom II programme running from 1997 to 2000. MedCom II has three goals:
- dissemination of the communication of the classical information flows;
- developing communication in home-care area;
- establishing new pilot projects in new areas in regional health: Internet, tele-medicine and tele-consulting.

4.3.6.2 Dissemination

In the period towards year 2000, regional dissemination projects are going to ensure rapid and massive dissemination of the use of communication standards developed in the period 1994-96. The goal is to reach 22 million messages, or 68% of the total communication in regional healthcare, before year 2000. As a part of this effort, all Danish counties have made their own exploitation plans for each of the classical information flows in healthcare, and set a regional target for the dissemination in the region by year 2000.

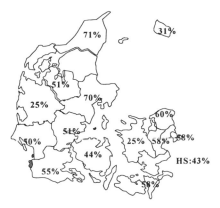

Figure 14: Goal for the total communication in Danish RHCNs by 1999

4.3.6.3 Home care

Besides dissemination, a number of information flows should be developed specially for the municipal area through a number of pilot projects involving home care and social security in the local authorities, hospitals, pharmacies etc. The home-care area is working with communication to and from hospitals in connection with hospital treatment, especially for elderly people, and is developing standards for clinical protocols concerning maternity co-operation between hospitals, home care, social care and GPs.

4.3.6.4 New pilots

To test new sorts of communication in a RHCN concerning images, the use of Internet, tele-medicine and tele-consulting, a series of minor pilot projects are planned. The largest of these is a dental project, setting up a regional network between dentists, hospitals, universities and dental laboratories with the focus on tele-medicine and tele-consulting. Another project, MedCity, is working on creating a health-city, where many different parties are using many different tools with the goal of communicating all information electronically.

4.4   Finland

4.4.1   Healthcare organisation

Finland is divided into 21 hospital districts owned by the local municipal authorities. Most districts have 2-3 hospitals covering from 100.000 - 800.000 inhabitants. In five regions, there is a university hospital. Every local municipal authority has its own health centre where GPs work. Many health centres have investigation services of their own.

Finland has public healthcare paid by taxes, with equal access to healthcare for all citizens irrespective of where they live or how much they earn. Since 1993, the community in which the person resides is responsible for arranging for the availability of healthcare services, and for paying for these services. GPs in the primary health centres act as the gatekeepers to specialised care.

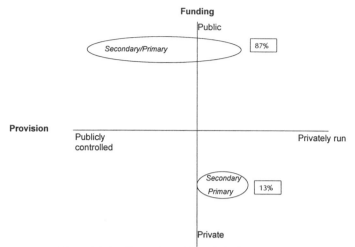

Figure 15: Funding and provision of Finnish healthcare

Patients can also elect to use private sector services. Private sector physicians can refer patients to specialised care in the public sector. The cost is financed through a combination of communal taxes, state taxes, the national health insurance plan, and, in some cases, patient part-contributions.

4.4.2   Information flows

Almost all communications in healthcare in Finland are regional: between the hospitals in the region, and between hospitals and GPs. Only a minor part crosses regional borders between local hospitals and national university hospitals - and almost no communication crosses national borders.

Most of the communication is textual, covering the classical information flows such as prescriptions, laboratory results and so on. This communication is normally done by ordinary mail, or else by local parcel services set up in larger cities gathering laboratory requests or prescriptions. There is little communication of images and pictures. Consultation with experts is not normally organised formally, but ad-hoc phone calls from GPs to hospitals are used instead.

4.4.3   IT systems in healthcare

In Finland, all hospitals use Patient Administration Systems, and other systems for investigation services. Most hospitals have significant networking capability, while EDI messages are coming into widespread use. A wide consensus exists on migration towards systems integration, open interfaces (APIs) and object orientation. There are few regional programmes for introducing Electronic Health Care Records (EHCR) in hospitals.

Almost all GPs (80%) have implemented IT systems.

IT Providers

About 10 different IT providers offer IT solution to Finnish healthcare. In the hospital area there are four different companies, and in primary care six different companies.

4.4.4   Current status of RHCN

In Finland there are a few concrete regional projects. The North Karelia Hospital District has developed an intelligent referral and electronic patient record, both of which are in the testing phase. The intelligent referral will be in daily use in 1999 in 13 different health centres and two hospitals.

In Kymenlaakso Hospital District, they have a referral system based on e- mail. Also in Oulu region they have an electronic referral system and patient record system in the testing phase.

The Satakunta Macro Pilot is seeking to develop new services for health and social services. Macro Pilot seeks to develop services at a personal level by the use of new technologies among other methods.

The primary goal is to develop seamless services, which means that clients will receive a minimum of "run-around" by making relevant information more available.

Another goal is to improve the ability of citizens to be served in their homes. Information is to be moved electronically whenever possible. Information and client services focused on the citizen will make this possible. If the client does not possess the ability or opportunity to use them, s/he can authorise a social work healthcare professional to manage the information on his/her behalf. In Macro Pilot project this is called "case manager model".

Satakunta Macro Pilot will last to the end of the year 2000. During that time we will complete dozens of projects related to seamless service, independent access, information and client services and information confidentiality. There will be hundreds of professionals from different areas involved. At this time, projects underway or in the planning phase include:

- the planning of seamless care and service chains;
- support for independent access;
- case manager model;
- information and customer service;
- client identification card project;
- order and results of laboratory tests messaging between the Central Hospital and local health care clinics;
- social work and healthcare co-operation network;
- region-wide data security and protection;
- occupational health and safety protection development;
- regional care and service chain co-ordination, etc.

4.4.5   Industry - companies, products and services for RHCN

Almost all IT providers and especially tele-operators have solutions for communication of the classical information flows such as prescriptions, laboratory results etc.

Also some companies have developed general web-based information systems to support citizens and GPs in getting information from hospitals etc.

4.4.6   Future development of RHCN, 1998 - 2002

In Finland, some regions are developing RHCNs on a large scale. The focus will be on collaboration between hospitals and health centres, and in electronic referral patterns. The Ministry of Social Affairs and Health strongly supports the development of RHCNs in Finland.

The North Karelia Hospital District currently has plans for developing a RHCN. For the first phase, they are developing an intelligent electronic referral; this is in pilot phase just now. The Satakunta Macro Pilot, Kymenlaakso region and Oulu region also have regional plans and projects. Many of them are in testing phase, and will come into daily use in 2000.

The Ministry of Social Affairs and Health has published a strategy for IT at national level. In 2-4 years, many projects will develop RHCN systems in Finland, and also many regions will use them.

Compared to most of the rest of Europe, Finland is a very sparsely populated country. Tele-medicine has excellent potential to realise a model where the GP or other healthcare professional working in the front line of care delivery can be supported by specialist clinicians at centres of excellence. This type of virtual hospital is a reality already in some healthcare domains.

In many sparsely populated counties, tele-medicine is seen as the means of saving many small health centres from closing down. It gives the GP or other health professional working in a remote location much needed professional support in terms of second opinion and access to continuous medical education. For the national strategy, probably the major benefit from tele-medicine is the ability to get top level expertise offered in a local surgery, or even at home, and the possibility of competition between the units offering specialised services.

4.5   France

4.5.1   Healthcare organisation

Healthcare in France is organised in a different way from other European countries, and French citizens are very proud of their social security system, although it is often a nightmare to balance the accounts. The system is unique due to the importance of the private sector, and also due to the complete freedom given to citizens to consult any physician (GP, specialist etc.). Recently, the Ministry of Health has introduced a new organisation called "médecin référent", in which a citizen agrees to consult always the same GP, who would then act as a gatekeeper responsible for referring the patient to secondary care and keeping the patient's electronic file.

In France there are two major political/administrative levels: the central government and the regional level.

The Ministry of Employment and Solidarity is responsible for defining the general policy in healthcare, the social insurance budget and the social objectives. It draws up terms of reference and prepares government regulations. It is further divided into several secretariats - one of these is dedicated to healthcare issues.

Special departments have been created to take charge of specific issues regarding the various tasks to be carried out.

- The General Board of Health (Direction Générale de la Santé) - This is the government's central advisory agency in the field of health care. The key task of this agency is to evaluate the services provided in order to see whether they correspond to the population needs and then to define suitable healthcare policies.

- The General Board for Hospital (Direction des Hôpitaux) - This is in charge of the budgetary repartition for the overall secondary and tertiary care. It has to work in co-ordination with all the regional agencies (ARH) in order to be able to evaluate the specific regional needs.

- The General Board of Social Security (Direction de la Sécurité Sociale) - This agency is in charge of the management of social security, which is the main system of social insurance. It has to guarantee that the system is well suited to carry out its missions, and it has to find the means for funding. One of its main missions to take charge of the reimbursement of the care expenditure of the population; another major one is to negotiate the activities and the incomes of the primary care actors.

Various agencies with regional responsibility exist:

- The Regional Agency for Hospital (ARH) - The agency is commissioned to set, at a regional level, the government policy. In a competitive environment, and as far as possible, it has to co-ordinate the different healthcare enterprises in terms of activities, and determine an agreed level of funding for each hospital. Institutional representatives of the ARH work together with the healthcare professionals.

- The Regional committees: DRASS and DASS - These regional committees group political and healthcare professional representatives, and are responsible for observation, analysis and the definition of priorities in terms of social and healthcare issues at the regional level. They are members of the executive committees of the Regional Agencies for Hospital (ARH).

Hospitals are in principle paid on the basis of PMSI (Programme de Médicalisation des Systèmes d'Information), itself being based on Diagnosis Related Groups (DRGs). To administer this, a new department has been created within the hospitals called DIM (Département d'Information Médicale), even if the system has not been deployed to its full extent, and some readjustments to iron away losses are still common practice. The PMSI is the first step in the accreditation process. Hospitals and clinics have to be equipped with an information system which allow the entry and reporting of the necessary information required by the programme.

There are 3419 hospitals in France (the biggest number after Germany), which represent 564.000 beds. The hospital equipment is 10,1 beds per 1.000 inhabitants. They are classified as hospital group institutions (Assistance Publique Paris, Marseille, Hospices Civils de Lyon), Regional Hospital Centres, General Hospital Centres, Dedicated Hospital Centres and Local Hospitals.

Physicians of the private sector (GPs, Specialists, Clinics etc...) are independent professionals bound by their convention (see above), and are remunerated according to the number and type of acts performed for which they may charge their own rates. Patients have to report to social security (sending social security forms) to get reimbursed. In 1996, Prime Minister Juppé launched the Sesam-Vitale programme to create direct electronic communications between physicians and social security centres. There are about 100,000 private medical doctors in France (including the specialist doctors).

The authorities are trying to push organisation schemas able to provide continuity of care. This is one of the reasons for the launching of the "médecin référent" system and the RSS (Réseau Santé Social, see below).

The budget of the system is funded by general taxation on salaries ("charges sociales") and may be topped-up if necessary by the public treasury. In principle, citizens still have to pay a part of the cost ("ticket modérateur"), except if they are classified in a different way due to their illness or their social situation. The private sector is bound by so-called "conventions" (contracts, negotiated at national level); some of them allow the physician to charge whatever rates they like, but the patient is only reimbursed the same fee by social security. Very recently, for the first time some physicians have been taxed because social security considered that their rates were too high, since they did not deliver exceptional services; this was in opposition to the objective of granting the same access to health for all citizens. The level of coverage of social security depends on the type of healthcare service (large surgery interventions are covered 100%, with small medications covered 66%, while some others are not covered at all). People may contract with private health insurers (Mutuelles) in order to be secured for the complementary part.

People usually have to pay in advance and ask for reimbursement, except if the process called "tiers-payant" applies.

The reimbursement obtained by public + private insurance may still not be complete in some circumstances.

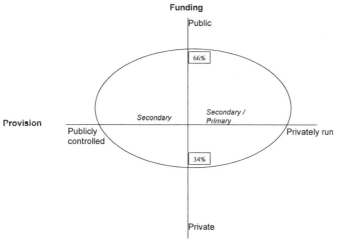

Figure 16: Funding and provision of French healthcare

With respect to control of health care delivery, most large hospitals are public and provide secondary care, although it is possible for citizens to consult directly without going through a GP. People can also choose their GP or specialist at any time (freedom of choice very important for French citizens). Recently the reform of "médecin référent" provides an additional possibility, citizens contracting with their GP and thereby abandoning their freedom of choice.

Specialists may work in public hospitals or in private hospitals or clinics or in their private "cabinet". GP work in their private "cabinet", sometimes in association with other GPs.

In summary, in France every permutation is possible: private secondary care, public secondary care, public funding, private funding; the situation is evaluated case by case. Of course, the complexity of the system probably leads to important overheads.

4.5.2 Information flows

The classic system is exceptional in France and is related only to the new "médecin référent" organisation.

But in most of the cases, the clinical information flow consists of physicians wanting to get news of the care provided to their patient when in hospital and hospitals sending discharge letters.

In practice, and because the administration is a little better organised than the clinicians, most of the communications relates in administrative area: social security forms from private sector to social security, Standardised Discharge Summaries from public sector to DRASS, funds transfer related EDI messages etc.

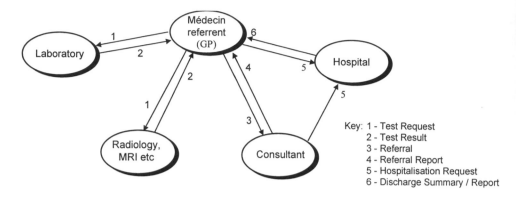

Figure 17: French "médecin référent" information flows

4.5.3 IT systems in healthcare

Primary Care

Due to the creation of the Sesam-Vitale system, healthcare professionals have been all of a sudden obliged to get equipped with an IT system. This includes computer, special card readers to read the Health Professional smart card and the patient smart card, and software conforming to social security specifications allowing to send electronic forms to social security. The system has met strong resistances from physicians' syndicates up to now, due to big mistakes in its organisation, but 80% of physicians might be equipped at the end of 1999. The equipment cost will be partly funded by the government and social security.

Primary Care Information Systems

Due to Sesam-Vitale, there have been many new providers of medical record software for primary care, including tele-transmission facilities. An extract of the list is provided in Table 1 below. There are about 100,000 physicians to equip.

Table 10: Primary Care Information Systems Suppliers

ADAMIS	Eglantine Informatique	Ordosoft
ADSM Informatique	HATIS	PLEXUS
Alcatel	HDMP	POLYTEL
Alternative Soft	ICSF	SAPHIS
BIOSTAT	Imagine Editions	SETE AXILOG
Cequoia Concept	Instar Informatique	Shared Medical Systems
COCCILOG SA	LSI Médical	SIAMUC - SIAMED
DISTAL	MEDCOM	Societe Intersysteme
Easylogique	MICRO 6	VARIMED
EBP	NW Soft	01 SANTE SA

Very few of these follow the work of the European standardisation bodies related to EHCR (Env 12265 and follow-up standards).

Secondary Care

The computerisation of hospitals has started, as in any other country, with the administrative systems, followed by a variety of departmental systems addressing only the specific needs of a clinical service. Only recently has the need to share information and to integrate these islands of IT with one another become apparent. Current Invitations to Tender favour integrated solutions to be implemented from scratch, or solutions based on integration middleware, which allow hospitals, within certain limits, to retain the existing departmental systems. The first of them (REFERENCE) was an outcome of the European RICHE Esprit project, and was very nearly pushed towards all hospitals by the government (the decision was even publicly announced by the authorities). Due to the pressure of competitors of CAP-Gemini and Bull (involved in REFERENCE), the authorities had to pull back and now promote solutions based on the European pre-standard architecture for Health Information Systems (HISA). Decisions are taken at individual hospital level after calls for tenders.

IT networks are present in more than 80% of hospital centres and in all regional hospital centres. Mainly they are conventional networks: only 16% of hospital centres own a high speed network (52% for Regional Hospital Centres). TCP/IP is widely spread (100% of Regional Hospital Centres, 66% of Hospital Centres, 80% of Dedicated Hospital Centres); it is also used in the RSS.

56% of hospitals have permanent IT links with one or more external organisations (networks open towards the external world: 84% of Regional Hospital Centres, 53% of Hospital Centres and 60% of Dedicated Hospital Centres).

Access to Internet is still low (31% of Hospitals, 77% of Regional Health Centres, 29% of Hospital Centres and 26% of Dedicated Hospital Centres) but should grow rapidly.

Most hospitals already exchange information with other organisations (treasuries, payment bodies etc...). 61% of Regional Health Centres participate, 55% of Hospital Centres and 54% of Dedicated Hospital Centres.

The areas where IT systems are most common are:
- administrative (accounting, stock control, payroll) - 90%;
- laboratory departments - 71%;
- pharmacy - 67%.

Clinical activities are supported by IT only in 48%, and diagnostic departments (imaging) in 38%; operating theatres are even lower at 23%.

Hospital Information Systems

Hospital Information Systems have been traditionally organised through solutions for hospital groups, for example SIR, STAF, Mediane, Symphonie, C-Page, Profils.

The new generation of solutions, which address clinical information and executive information requirements, is based on open systems and is increasingly offered over client-server architectures with graphical user interface.

The leading edge products are designed around industry specific middleware (REFERENCE, SYMPHONIE, C-PAGE), which represent the glue allowing heterogeneous departmental applications to share databases, exchange data and provide services to one another.

Cap-Gemini is the promoter of the REFERENCE solutions.

Most of the other groups are still organised as public groupings of IT resources.

Bull has still the most important share of the market due to its historic advantage as a public company.

Kalamazoo has made some good progress in the recent years with small size hospitals.

SMS is also entering the French market, and is gaining market share in France. It has recently acquired Pyrénees-Informatique, which is the leader in the clinic sector.

In addition, there are many SMEs providing specific software on top of the kernels provided by the big groups. This includes organisations like SIB (Syndicat Interhospitalier de Bretagne), Cecosi (PMSI software), SAPHIS (EHCR software) etc.

Big companies like Thompson or Alcatel also provides dedicated solutions, mainly as integrators.

4.5.4   Current status of RHCN

The French authorities wish to create a national network for healthcare and social care. Réseau Santé Social (RSS). It is wished to be able to federate all other related networks, fast and secure, and dedicated to healthcare and social care professionals

After a call for tender, CEGETEL offer was accepted for 5 years.

The RSS is supposed to grant to all healthcare professionals a secured space for communication, exchanging information, data, images, sharing knowledge, in a simple and efficient way.

In addition, other service providers might offer new applications and propose value added services to healthcare professionals. These services shall be agreed first by public authorities and have to conform to strict confidentiality and ethical constraints.

The RSS is based on Internet technologies, offering in a secure way a gateway to the world wide web.

The main domains of use of the RSS are:

- Secure information exchange between users:
  - Patient related information allowing better care and disease management, and co-ordination of care between the different healthcare actors. These exchanges will permit a more efficient communication between primary care and secondary care. In addition, they will accelerate and simplify some daily exchanges such as laboratory reports.

- Anonymous information such as reports related to activities of healthcare professionals or various statistics.
- Public health alert information, for example to follow up the spread of an epidemic.

- Access to documentation and reference material:
    - Medical publications, databases, guidelines etc.
    - Training services, quality assurance information, diagnostic support, prescription support, clinical trials etc.

The main services provided by the RSS are:
- authentication of users;
- mailbox system within the RSS and with Internet users;
- users and services diaries;
- connection toolkits;
- secure information exchange space for physicians;
- transmission of Social Security forms;
- Internet access;
- customer assistance;
- other value-added services provided by service providers.

The RSS started officially in the Brittany area on 2nd April 1998. There are now about 35 departments covered, but only some dozens of physicians connected. There will soon be an evolution in the cryptographic services used, including S/MIME 40 bits.

4.5.5 Industry - companies, products and services for RHCN

Networks for Healthcare

Due to the recent developments (Sesam-Vitale, RSS), several networks are under development due to private initiatives. The physicians syndicates have launched their own networks (Medsyn, SIAMUC).

Regional Unions of Physicians would like to do the same.

Complementary insurance and pharmaceutical industry looking at Disease Management are also involved in the development of complementary networks.

Those networks would be connected to the RSS as shown in Figure 18 below.

The main industrial actors are CEGETEL, France Telecom, Alcatel, medical record software providers, hospital systems providers etc.

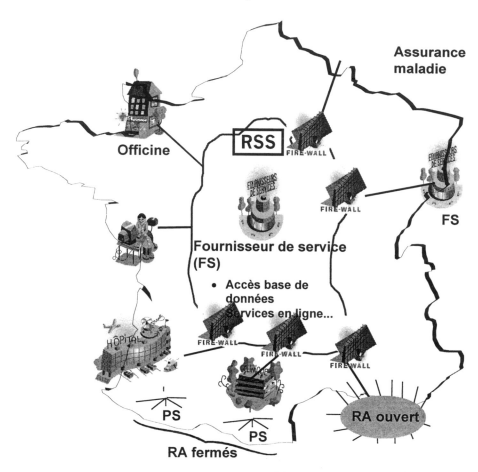

Figure 18: RSS network in France

4.5.6   Future development of RHCN, 1998 - 2002

The main driving forces towards healthcare networks (but not necessarily regional) in France are:

- the deployment of Sesam-Vitale;

- the deployment of the RSS;

- political constraints, such as the necessity for physicians to build their own networks in order to gather as much information as social security, so they can better negotiate the conventions with them;

- the setting up of regional organisations, like ARH (Agence Regionale d'Hospitalisations) and URML (Unions Régionales de Médecins Libéraux);

- the growing interest from the health insurance and pharmaceutical industries for medical information.

Most of the networks already working concern tele-medicine applications, most of them being communication of images to a specialist consultants and discussion of a particular medical case.

These kinds of networks tend to grow, and are usually disconnected from other types of networks.

New networks will probably first concern private initiatives, like the network of South-west area (Moselle-Est, Eure et Loir, Limousin). They will mainly address concentration of social security forms in order to create detailed statistics for better managed care and better negotiations with public authorities.

Most of these networks will be linked with the RSS, as was presented in a previous section.

There will be scientific networks addressing particular problems, and disease management networks promoted by the health insurance or pharmaceutical industries.

In the frame of the Star project, SAPHIS has developed a solution for healthcare yellow pages services for healthcare professionals and citizens. This will allow them to select the medical service they need from all the potential providers established in the area, both public and private. This implies that they should be given a dynamic picture of the healthcare offering, including information about waiting time and price.

Most of these networks and services will have to evolve in liaison with the RSS, which is supposed to be the main federating network. The services provided by the RSS have been already described in a previous section.

The main challenge will be related to interoperability of systems connected to these networks. It is not yet clear that the major actors have well understood the importance of standards in this area, and the specificity of healthcare and healthcare related information in relation to other sectors.

4.6   Germany

4.6.1   Healthcare organisation

Germany has both a public and a private insurance system which covers all necessary healthcare expenditures of citizens. Citizens with higher incomes or self-employed citizens can choose a private healthcare insurance. During the period 1994-98 there was a tendency to reduce the coverage of public insurance, and to cover more and more expense by private means.

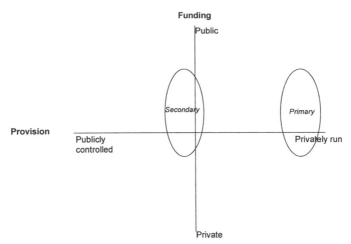

Figure 19: Funding and provision of German healthcare

Care is delivered by two complementary sectors: general and specialist ambulatory care practitioners, and the hospital sector (with only a marginal outpatient sector). Hospitals are about one-third publicly owned (mainly the larger hospitals), one-third private, and one-third church or other charitable organisations. The federal states are responsible for the provision of health care, under the provision of federal regulations. Significant changes are now coming about as a result of new federal regulations, designed to contain the increasing costs of health care, and also permitting hospitals to enlarge the outpatient sector, in particular by ambulant surgical care.

Healthcare service providers invoice public health insurance either directly (hospitals) or, in the case of primary care, via regional organisations called Kassenärztliche Vereinigungen (KV). In any case, these patients are not directly involved in the administrative reimbursement procedure. For citizens covered by private insurance, healthcare service providers invoice the patients who claim the expenses back form their insurance.

For all public healthcare expenses, the KV represents the clearing house and regulatory body for primary care institutions. (Primary care in Germany covers many special medical disciplines, such as paediatrics, orthopaedics, day case surgery etc. operated in ambulatory medical practices). As such, the regional scope of the KV defines the "natural" healthcare region. In Germany there are 23 such regions.

4.6.2 Information flows

Clinical information flows between healthcare providers in a region are as described at the start of this section.

The traditional and most important communication scenarios for exchange of administrative information within a region are illustrated by Figure 20.

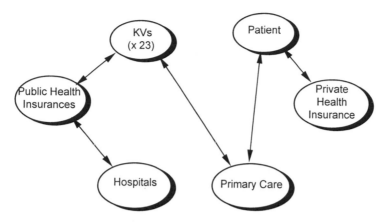

Figure 20: Typical administrative information flows in Germany

The majority of all transactions take place within the region; the major share is still handled via paper mail, phone or courier.

4.6.3   IT systems in healthcare

The national developments in RHCNs in Germany have been influenced strongly by political decisions. The law called Gesundheitsstrukturgesetz introduced a freeze of all public healthcare expenditures, for primary care, secondary care, drug prescriptions and rehabilitation. On the other hand, all the well known developments took place: growing demand for healthcare services, both in terms of quality and quantity, and rising operational costs. This situation led to a high degree of reluctance for all types of investments, including investments in IT. In practice, investments in this sector concentrated on IT infrastructure, where a clear benefit could be shown; this was the case primarily for administrative systems for primary care and in-house networking solutions for hospitals.

In 1993/4, a credit card sized electronic health insurance card was introduced for all customers of public insurance. It contains only basic data such as patient name, address, date of birth, sex and insurance company. Although there is more capacity, medical data is not allowed to be stored. At the beginning of 1998, 66% of primary care practices were equipped with PCs, in most cases forming small LANs of three to five systems; all primary care service providers are equipped with card readers and printers, which are needed to handle the electronic health insurance card.

Primary Care

In primary care IT systems are being used in the first instance to manage the quarterly invoice procedure to KVs and the very complex and always changing catalogue of services and their respective reimbursement. In addition, the time planning functions are often used. Only some doctors use the systems for systematic documentation, archiving of information or communication. Even if electronic documentation is being used, many doctors keep traditional paper based records in parallel; this is because of the uncertainties of the legal sustainability of an exclusive electronic archive of patient data.

Secondary Care

Hospital information systems are widely used for management and - with the exception of certain departmental areas - to a lesser degree for medical purposes. Laboratory management systems are commonplace, and computerised systems are used also in radiology, radiotherapy, and cardiology. Computers are also widely used for patient administration purposes including minimum basic data sets, discharge letters and operating theatre schedules.

4.6.4   Current status of RHCN

On the basis of the expectations raised by R&D projects in tele-medicine Europe-wide, a considerable number of tele-medicine and later on health telematics projects were started. However, due to a lack of realistic economical assessments, partially wrong technical concepts and the situation described above, there was no natural migration towards co-operative, cross-organisational IT networking structures. As in other parts of Europe, most projects were driven by technological enthusiasm and public funds, rather than by the real needs of users and economic or business considerations. Because of the political shift to market orientation of the healthcare system, the behaviour of sector actors is increasingly driven by competition rather than co-operation. So, as at the end of 1997, the use of healthcare telematics in Germany is concentrated on the following applications and services[15]:

- transfer of charging and billing data via diskette (66% of all ambulant doctors). There have been trials to transmit encrypted charging and billing data via data links; however, up until now this method has not made a break through;

- transfer of laboratory data;

- e-mail (2% of all doctors);

- use of on-line data bases (6% of all doctors);

- use of Internet (8% of all doctors).

Nevertheless, during 1994-98 there has been considerable progress in preparing the ground for the comprehensive and consequent use of healthcare telematics. This concerns basically standards and legislation.

The following standards have been released:

- ADT - Abrechnungsdatenträger: a standard describing interface and data sets for charging services from primary care institutions to public health insurance.

- BDT - Behandlungsdatenträger: a standard describing the interface of administrative IT systems for primary care institutions (Praxis EDV) and data sets of patient records (examinations, findings, treatment). This standard was defined to allow an exchange of administrative data, however it also allows the exchange of patient data.

- LDT - Labordatenträger: a standard describing laboratory data.

- Encryption module: allows symmetric encryption of data and will become mandatory for use of ADT, LDT, BDT, etc.

- HL7: nearly 100% use of HL7 in hospitals.

- ICD9/10: ICD codification of diseases is mandatory in hospitals; trials to impose the use of ICD in primary care have not been successful so far.

The legal situation with regard to electronic patient records and communication of patient data is being clarified:

- Major issues implied by the Information Society have been ruled by the Informations und Kommunikationsdienstegesetz[16]. This law and subsequent regulations put the many healthcare telematics applications legally on safe ground, e.g. the communication of patient data and tele-archiving, or the archiving of x-ray and CT-images exclusively in electronic form[17].

At the end of 1998, there are not many providers of services in Germany which go beyond "content only" service providers. At the moment there is only Deutsche Telekom with its service "Global Health Care"[i] (GHC), a dedicated intranet solution for the healthcare sector. The service can be accessed locally throughout Germany via standard browsers, and addresses all groups of users from professionals to citizens. GHC has a layered security concept. The highest level comes with chip card based access control, user authentication, encryption and electronic signature, illustrated by Figure 21.

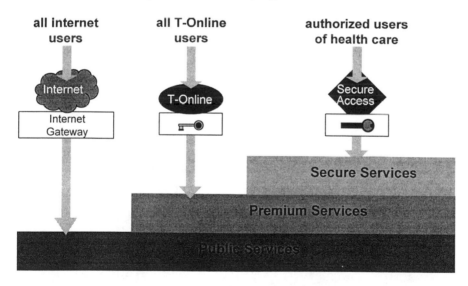

Figure 21: Services and access concepts of Global Health Care

"Public Services" are accessible via internet or T-Online® and cover
- all types of public healthcare information in a structured way;
- access to internet;

---

i   Global Health Care, GHC, for further information see http://www.telekom.de/angebot/

- all services and information of T-Online, one of the largest general on-line services.

The service is designed to address the needs of citizens and patients and is planned to be accessible by end 1998.

The "Premium Service" is accessible via T-Online; access is controlled, and the service supports billing functions for content providers. Subscribers pay a monthly fee and content providers can charge users for accessing the information. The content offered covers:
- special information, e.g. access to databases, on-line books etc.;
- educational information;
- e-commerce (internet shopping etc.);
- on-line banking.

For content providers it is an on-line market place for marketing and sales.

The last offering, "Secure Service", addresses the needs of professionals with regard to communication of confidential data and covers two services: "Secure Mail" and "Secure Web". The service provides Secure Mail communication for all types of confidential information such as patient or charging/billing data. Subscribers receive, besides a software package, a chip card and a chip card reader. The chip card, issued by a trusted centre, contains the private electronic key of the subscriber (1024 bit) and hence the digital signature of the owner. Messages are encrypted using the public key method. Beside Secure Mail, there will be the possibility to use Secure Web services, which enable hospitals or other medical content providers to publish confidential information via Web server. Access is controlled similarly to Secure Mail. Secure Web will be available at the end of 1998. All service products are consistent with the strict data protection legislation of Germany. Figure 22 illustrates the various service and security features of GHC.

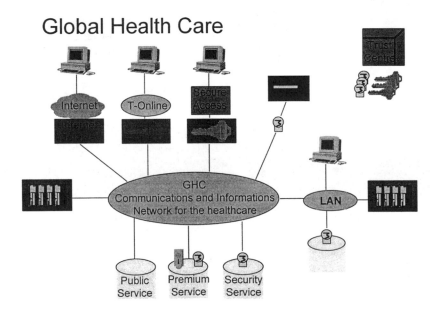

Figure 22: Service and security features of Global Health Care

Beside Deutsche Telekom there is the Deutsches Gesundheitsnetz[j] (DGN), operated by o-tel-o, one of the new operators of telecommunication services in Germany. The offer of DGN covers (mid 1998):

- internet access,
- e-mail,
- access to medical data bases,
- on-line banking.

The network represents an intranet with its own regional access points for major cities. Access is controlled; the support of asymmetric encryption techniques is planned. The network is planned to be extended step by step. DGN managed to liaise with a number of regional healthcare administrative institutions (Kassenaerztliche Vereinigungen, Ärztekammern) who publish their information via DGN.

By mid 1998, there are no other operators of RHCN services providing a complete product and service offering, who are active on a country-wide scale. However, there are several regional projects and initiatives implementing specific healthcare telematics supported medical corporations. In many cases these activities are project based and driven by research or public interests, and their broader acceptance and economical viability remains to be seen.

In addition to the RHCN operators, there are many "content-only" medical on-line service providers (own content and web-hosting) who represent major assets for the on-line scene with regard to special information, education and health administrative information. Some operators provide free access, mostly run by pharmaceutical industries, others require subscription with monthly fees. Among the free on-line services there are many semi-professional services. The main problem with this group is that their information is often not up-to-date. The number of services is growing and the actors are changing. A good up-to-date overview can be found in journals such as Medonline[18] or Praxis-Computer[19].

Major professional medical "content-only" on-line service providers at the end of 1998 in Germany are shown in the following table:

Table 11: On-line service providers in Germany

On-line Service	Operator	URL
Medworld	Boehringer Ingelheim Pharma	http://medworld.de
SB-Online	SmithKline Beacham Pharma	http://www.sb-online.de
multimedica	Health Online Service, Berlin (Burda)	http://www.multimedica.de/

Beside the services above there are a growing number of regional healthcare institutions present in the Web whose focus is more on the regional issues and therefore of particular relevance.

---

j   Deutsches Gesundheitsnetz, DGN, for further information see http://www.dgn.de

4.6.5 Industry - companies, products and services for RHCN

In Germany there are many companies active in areas relevant in one way or another to RHCN. In general it is recommended to attend special fairs to get the up-to-date information for the specific fields of interest. In Germany there is for example MEDICA, the world's largest fair of its kind covering all aspects of infrastructure and services for healthcare service operators, including components for.

Table 12: IT system suppliers in Germany

IT-systems	Companies.
Tele-Medicine Systems: Tele-Radiology, Tele-Pathology, Archiving	Deutsche Telekom (Tele-radiology Systems), Mediagate (central archiving, www.mediagate.de), Zeiss,
Administrative systems[k] including EHCR for Primary Care	Albis, CompuMED, Data-Vital, DOCexpert, Frey, Medistar, MCS, promedico, Sysmed Süd-West, Turbomed, ...
RHCN-VANS / Tele-operators in HC	Deutsches Gesundheitsnetz (DGN), Deutsche Telekom AG: (Global Healthcare), Medical Data Service GmbH
Medical On-line services	Deutsche Telekom (Global Health Care - On-line Service for medical professionals), Deutsches GesundheitsNetz (DGN) (o-tel-o,), HOS (Health On-line Service) http://www.dgn.de, Multimedica
Organisations	Medical Network e.V.

The Table 12 shows a subset of healthcare IT providers and organisations which are of particular relevance for RHCNs. The table is necessarily incomplete, while the sequence does not imply a ranking.

4.6.6 Future development of RHCN, 1998 - 2002

The period before 1998 was (as in the EU in general) very much determined by technological enthusiasm with regard to health telematics. It took a few years to map the things technically feasible with user needs and economical feasibility. The products described in section 3.1 have their roots in various national and international R&D activities. In the case of global healthcare, essential impact came from EU co-funded programmes such as AIM[l] and Telematics for Health[m], e.g. from projects like CHIN. The products can be seen as the result of a development, demonstration and validation process, and represent true innovations, because the products are based on inventions which survived the difficult process of serious business planning.

On a political level, it is generally recognised in Germany that health telematics and RHCNs can provide a dramatic improvement of the healthcare system as a whole. There is,

---

k KBV-Statistik Praxis-EDV: top ten in systems sold between January 1, 1997 – September 30, 1997
l Advanced Informatics in Medicine, Research Framework Programme III, 1991 -1994
m Research Framework Programme IV, 1995 -1998

for example, the "forum info 2000", working group 7[n]: "Telematik-Anwendung im Gesundheitswesen", initiated by the German federal ministry of health, which gathers leading representatives of medical organisations, health administrations and IT industry. This forum is aimed at the discussion of the implications and potential of the information society in healthcare, and at the production of recommendations and guidelines for the development, implementation and operation of IT&T technologies in the healthcare sector.

There is on the one hand an increase in political awareness of the potential of RHCNs and a willingness to support them, and on the other hand a growing economical pressure to save resources wherever possible. It is therefore realistic to forecast that the scope and coverage of the emerging RHCN products will be extended during the next years. There were in 1998 a few healthcare districts in Germany who supported trials called Vernetzte Praxen, a type of healthcare telematics assisted co-operation of independent practices. The healthcare districts (KV) provide some financial benefits for participants of the co-operation. It can be expected that this type of regional healthcare telematics structure will prosper. However, it is also clear that, at least in countries with a larger share of private medical service providers like Germany, investment will always be driven by organisation-specific economic considerations, rather than general health arguments. In addition, the "forum info 2000" clearly stated that in Germany there are severe barriers to the countrywide and harmonised implementation of RHCN. These barriers are:

- Organisation: The German healthcare system is a decentralised system under control of non-profit and non-governmental regional organisations. This structure implies that there is no central body who can "impose" rules or guidelines easily. All agreements are the result of a democratic decision making process. This generates additional problems with regard to extended RHCN structures, which should be compatible, at least in one country. Furthermore, there is no general programme that fosters the introduction of healthcare telematics in a structured, scientific and co-ordinated way. Info 2000 is the first attempt into this direction; the impact of the forum remains to be seen. Furthermore, as the consequent introduction of healthcare telematics will have drastic implications on the healthcare organisations, there are many actors who are hesitant to support developments that may lead to a change of hierarchies and long established organisational structures.

- Data protection/security: There has been considerable progress with respect to the legal basis in electronic archiving of patient data and communicating sensitive data using public networks; this has been discussed in more detail above. However, there is still no general mandatory recommendation or guideline with regard to infrastructures and operational processes required to guarantee the level of security which is legally required.

- Standardisation: There are many standards in place which allow inter-institutional communication on a case by case basis; this has been discussed in more detail above. However, the standards xDT used in the primary care sector are (as is the case with other standards) not a guarantee that one vendor's IT system can communicate with another vendor's without a

---

n   http://www.forum-info2000.de/Forum_Info_2000/Vorstellung-Menu.html
    http://www.forum-info2000.de/Links/AG7.html

problem. In addition, hospitals use HL7 coded data, but this is incompatible with xDT; hence there is a problem in communication between hospitals and the primary care sector.

- Motivation of users: From a user's perspective, it is difficult to find arguments to invest in RHCN or to subscribe to them. In the light of the shrinking income of medical professionals, investments are planned very carefully. As long as the barriers mentioned above exist, with no convincing economic arguments for participating in medical co-operation supported by healthcare telematics, the use of RHCN structures will remain limited to the use of internet and subscription to the content-only type of healthcare on-line services.

- User demands, costs of medical innovations and frozen budgets for healthcare services: The situation, described in more detail above, is not overcome. The unavoidable competition between healthcare service providers is not a good ground for any kind of co-operative structure.

4.7   *Ireland*

4.7.1   Healthcare organisation

Regional health boards administer the health services in Ireland. These agencies are responsible for the delivery of both healthcare and personal social services in their geographic region. There are eight such regions in the country ranging in population size between 250.000 - 1.200.000 people.

Each Board is responsible for providing a range of both health and personal social services in its geographic region; it administers healthcare services in its area, and is responsible for hospital, community and primary care sectors. These Boards are made up of representatives from: local authorities (local politicians), elected nominees from certain health professions, and a number of ministerial appointments.

The Department of Health is primarily concerned with policy matters, funding, and evaluation at national level. While some income is generated at local level, funding is mostly provided through the Department of Health from central taxation.

Not everyone is eligible for services 'free of charge'. Almost 40% of the population are medical cardholders entitled to a full range of health services without charge. They are defined as persons who are unable without undue hardship to arrange medical services (including GP and pharmacy) for themselves These people are registered with a GP. Eligibility for this service category is largely but not entirely or exclusively based on income.

The rest of the population (non-medical card holders) are entitled to free hospital services, apart from some nominal maintenance charges, but must pay privately for GP and pharmacy services. People in this category are not registered with a GP and are free to move between different practices. GPs are not employed directly by Health Boards but have a contract of service in respect of medical cardholders.

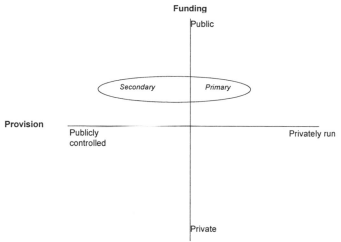

Figure 23: Funding and provision of Irish healthcare

Almost 40% of the population have private medical insurance which they can use to avail themselves of private treatment. Most public hospitals also offer private facilities. Hospital consultants provide both private and public services.

While many services are provided directly by Health Boards, some are delivered by voluntary agencies, which do not come under the control of Health Boards. Almost 50% of acute hospitals, and the majority of physical/mental handicap care, fall into this category. Currently these agencies are funded directly through central taxation but there are plans to change this arrangement.

Health Board services encompass both medical and non-medical areas. This presents opportunities for closer integration that might not exist in an alternative structure.

Referrals to hospitals are mostly through the GP service. Diagnostic facilities for GPs are normally provided by local hospitals.

In 1994 the government introduced a new strategy for the health services - 'Shaping a healthier future' - which sets down the clear objectives of achieving health and social gain for the population. Health gain aims to improve health status, while social gain is concerned with the broader quality of life factors. The key principles that underpin the strategy are equity, quality of service and accountability. The new focus on accountability that has been enshrined in legislation seeks to give decision makers at all levels a clear understanding of their objectives and a responsibility for achieving them.

4.7.2 Information flows

Communications between GPs and hospitals cover the traditional items such as referrals, bookings, diagnostic requests, results reporting and discharge letters. This is still mostly paper based. A number of pilot projects are in place for the development of electronic links between primary and secondary care providers. In 1997, the Department of Health established a project with a view to agreeing standard approaches between participants at national level

A significant area of communication exists between the national payments agency - the GMS (Payments) Board - and GPs/Pharmacists. This currently involves high volume paper transactions that lend themselves to an electronic approach. A project to examine this whole area is ongoing.

Communications are not always confined within a region. Certain units operate as centres for national specialities, but most service units have loosely defined regional catchment areas. Boundaries are informal and not strictly adhered to. Patients are generally free to attend their unit/hospital of choice; this includes GP services. In urban areas with a greater variety and level of facilities, many patients are referred from outside a unit's catchment area.

4.7.3   IT systems in healthcare

Information systems have been long established and well advanced in most hospitals in Ireland. Departmental systems including laboratory, radiology and pharmacy are also in use in all the main hospitals. In primary care there have been initiatives for both GPs and pharmacies. One of the targets of the health strategy was to have 80% of GPs computerised by the end of 1998; most Health Boards have already achieved this.

IT Providers

It is policy in most regions to use 'off the shelf' IT products as much as possible. In most cases, hospital systems are provided by some of the major international suppliers. The Department of Health has also arranged for the development of a local system that is owned by the health sector. In recent years there has been a move towards using 'best of breed' for the different components of the total information system with the use of appropriate integration products.

Funding has been provided to support IT developments in primary care. An accreditation process has been put in place for primary care systems. There are about five main products that GPs tend to opt for. Nearly all pharmacies are computerised using systems from a small number of suppliers. Some regions have developed Intranets for GPs.

4.7.4   Current status of RHCN

Some regions use tele-medicine to overcome difficulties for patients due to their remoteness from centres of care.

One of the issues impeding the wider use of electronic communication is the lack of a national unique patient identifier. There are encouraging signs that this deficiency will soon be dealt with.

4.7.5   Industry - companies, products and services for RHCN

All regions have extensive Wide Area Networks in place to support business processes and data/voice communications. The main provider of the physical infrastructure is Telecom Eireann – the former state owned telecommunications provider. With the advent of de-regulation, alternative suppliers are becoming available. There are a wide range of sources for e-mail, Internet and other added value services. Some regions have established 'secure' environments for GPs and pharmacy communications.

4.7.6 Future development of RHCN, 1998 - 2002

The implementation of the health strategy "Shaping a healthier future" (1994) will require the development of enhanced health telematics. Information is identified as a key contributor to efficiency, effectiveness and quality in healthcare.

In the coming years, the expanding development and use of communication technologies throughout the wider community will also be reflected in regional healthcare developments. Current pilot projects will evolve into full-scale developed systems There will be significant investment in primary care telematics, with a particular emphasis on the automation of routine transaction based activities. Communication and data standards based on international norms will be applied. The demand for seamless care will force agencies to review business processes and exploit the opportunities that technology presents. Tele-medicine will underpin many service developments.

Many of the present hospital based information systems will have reached the end of their lifecycle. Although functionally rich and operationally effective, these products have their origins in a time when the technologies available were much less advanced than at present. Health agencies will therefore seek to avail themselves of modern products to replace the current generation of applications. There will be an emphasis on integration and integration tools. This will require integrated organisations, services and processes.

A national patient identifier can be expected. Patient systems using smart cards will be implemented.

Training and education in health telematics will grow. Clinical and service staff will become more involved in management issues, including the development of information systems.

4.8 Italy

4.8.1 Healthcare organisation

Healthcare finance in Italy relies on both general taxation and social insurance; however, although the vast majority of expenditure is financed through public money, a great deal of care is provided by the private sector. The relative importance of the private sector, compared with the public one, increases when moving from north to south, as a reflection of an uneven quality and efficiency of public structures over the national territory. In general though:

- For Primary care 100% of funding is public but the service is provided by independent contractors linked to NHS through a framework contract negotiated at both national and regional level.

- For Secondary care most of the funding (but not all) is public, while provision is a mix of public and private.

Chapter 4

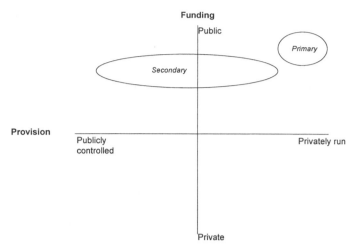

Figure 24: Funding and provision of Italian healthcare

Responsibility for healthcare delivery has been transferred from central government to regions over the last few years; each region is free, within broad limits, to organise itself the way it prefers to deliver services to citizens. The National Ministry of Health, however, still plays a major planning and controlling role; in particular, it is responsible for defining the minimum set of services any region has to guarantee to citizens.

The principle that the budget follows the patient is accepted in theory even if the information infrastructure to put the principle into practice is not yet in place. One of the hurdles to be overcome is caused by the identification of the patient: Italy does not have a unique health number for citizens. Alternatives such as the fiscal code (codice fiscale) are currently envisaged, but there is no general agreement about it, nor a legal obligation for patients to provide such a code to receive healthcare services.

The SSN (Italian National Health System) has undergone profound changes in the mid '90s, and the new organisational model is still subject to almost annual adjustments. The most important elements in the reorganisation of healthcare are territorial regrouping of USLs (Unità Sanitarie Locali - Local Health Units) and the establishment of ASLs (Aziende Sanitarie Locali - Local Health Authorities - LHA) and of Aziende Ospedaliere (Independently Managed Hospitals - IMH).

As a result of the regrouping (a reduction from the previous 674 Local Health Units to the present 223 Local Health Authorities), all the newly established LHAs cover a rather large area, normally corresponding to the Province, and include a vast and articulate network of hospital and community centres distributed across the territory.

In parallel, the 59 newly created Independently Managed Hospitals often constitute a single governing and management body for several hospital sites; these often have specific and differing specialities, and a geographical spread over the territory.

Moreover, all the LHAs have been granted considerable freedom to organise and manage themselves, within regional guidelines (which also vary widely from one region to another). This has created considerable variations in the structure, organisation and procedures of the different Authorities. In many cases also, the hospital sites reporting to the same LHA enjoy a high level of management freedom, causing potential significant differences within the Authority itself.

As well as the variety of structural and organisational models which have arisen, the reorganisation of healthcare has opened up ample opportunities for solutions based on co-operation between different structures (especially within the same LHA) which are a key factor in realising important economies of scale and management efficiencies.

In the private sector, the emphasis on competition implicit in the reorganisation has created a move towards wider use of the "multi-hospital system" formula, based on strong alliances between individual hospitals in a given territory, which result from both spontaneous collaboration and the creation of real private hospital networks.

Currently the SSN is organised into:
- Assessorati (Regional Health Authorities);
- ASL or USL (Local Health Authorities);
- Aziende Ospedaliere (Independently Managed Hospitals);
- GPs/Free Choice Paediatricians.

Social Services, on the contrary, are not under the responsibility of the SSN but are generally provided by municipalities. This makes the highly desirable co-ordination between health and social services rather difficult if not impossible.

Money to fund health expenditure is collected centrally and distributed to the regions according to their population and historic data. Regional Health Authorities, in turn, split the budget among the LHAs under their control, according to the same criteria. More accurate criteria based on age profile and epidemiological data are being discussed, to render the split more equitable.

Hospitals, on the contrary, are in principle paid on the basis of Diagnosis Related Groups (DRGs), even if the system has not been deployed to its full extent, and some readjustments to iron away losses are still common practice.

GPs and Free Choice Paediatrician are independent professionals linked to Local Health Authorities through a convention (contract), which is negotiated at national level first and at regional level later. GPs and Free Choice Paediatricians are basically remunerated according to capitation criteria, with a few acts, mostly administrative such as certificates, paid separately, directly by the patient.

Primary care is free of charge for all citizens, while outpatient consultations, drugs and some other secondary care services might require a financial contribution from the patient, unless the patient enjoys an exempted status due to financial (poverty) or health (serious and chronic diseases) conditions.

There is a growing trend towards a clearer separation between purchasing of healthcare and delivery of it, along the lines of the British model. The Italian way to the internal market for healthcare however differs from the British one in several respects:
- freedom of choice given to the patient;

- the prominent role of the private healthcare sector is seen as a real alternative to an "inefficient" public health service;
- absence of the fundholding concept.

This model has been pioneered already in 1998 by the Lombardia Region, without the previous approval by the central Ministry of Health; this has caused a serious rift between central and regional Government.

There is a clear push towards better integration between the different levels of care as the only adequate response to a demand for better quality and more affordable care. This mind set creates a very favourable environment for RHCNs.

Table 13: SSN organisation in Italy

Geographical Area	Northwest	Northeast	Centre	South	ITALY
ASLs	72	41	42	68	223°
Independently Managed Hospitals	25	7	12	9	53
General Practitioners	13,108	7,158	10,087	13,843	44,196
Free Choice Paediatricians	1,632	902	1,221	2,166	5,921

Total SSN spending for healthcare in 1997 was some 49 billion euros, which means 5.6% of Italian GNP, while spending on private health care is estimated at 20 billion euros.

4.8.2   Information flows

There are two principal categories of information flow:
- flows to support the clinical treatment of patients; these are standard, as described at the start of this section;
- flows to support the consolidation of health and administrative data at regional level. This latter flow will vary slightly from region to region, but it basically follows the scheme shown in Figure 25 below.

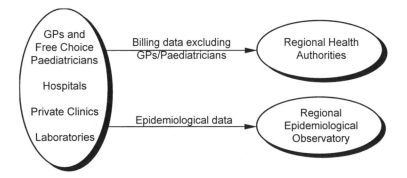

Figure 25: Epidemiological and administrative information flows in Italy

---

o   The number of ASLs is changing constantly as a result of a marked consolidation process which tends to increase their average size and decrease their number

4.8.3   IT systems in healthcare

Primary Care

The penetration of IT among GPs and Free Choice Paediatricians remains very low, because until now it has been left to the personal initiative of each individual health professional, with little or no encouragement at all from Health Authorities. It could be argued that the current 10-12% of GPs and Free Choice Paediatricians constitutes the ceiling for a spontaneous proliferation of IT within the profession.

The next wave of computerisation will only come about as a result of the deployment of RHCNs, of which the GP information system represents one of the main sources of data.

In this new context, the computerisation of GPs will be completely funded, or at least heavily subsidised, by the ASLs, who are the main beneficiaries of the rationalisation achieved through proper management and integration of health information in their territory.

Primary Care Information Systems

The largest supplier is PROFIM, a company based in Southern Italy and using a large publishing house, UTET, as its main sales channel. PROFIM's installed base is about 4.500 licences. Only three other products have gone past the 1.000 licences mark, MilleWin, Phronesis and Venere. MilleWin, in particular, enjoys the backing of SIMG, the Italian Scientific Association of General Medicine. None of these products is designed to support telematic links.

Telematics features are on the contrary present in two products which have the merit of existing but which are not on sale to general public:
- FUS from Janssen-Cilag, which has been supplied until now in the context of the Frameworks pilot in Rho and which should become available shortly through a new partnership with a commercial company.
- Medidoc, a Belgian product from Datasoft Management, which has been adapted to Italian requirements in the context of REMEDES. For this latter product there is no distribution agreement in place to sell the product in Italy.

Secondary Care

The computerisation of hospitals has started, as in any other country, with the administrative systems, followed by a variety of departmental systems addressing only the specific needs of a clinical service. Only recently has the need to share information and to integrate these islands of IT with one another become apparent. Current Invitations to Tender favour integrated solutions to be implemented from scratch, or solutions based on integration middleware, which allow hospitals to keep, within certain limits, the existing departmental systems. Decisions are taken at individual hospital level with a typical value for individual orders in the range of 1 to 1.5 million euros.

As of today, virtually all hospitals have IT systems in support of some of their clinical activities, though the take-up of such systems in different areas varies. The areas where IT systems are most common are:

- administrative (accounting, stock control, payroll);
- ADT (admission, discharge, transfer);
- outpatient and inpatient booking;
- diagnostic departments (laboratory, pathology, radiology, blood transfusion centre);
- pharmacy.

In Italy, as a consequence of the high fragmentation of decision making in the healthcare system, there is little sign of an overall strategy concerning IT in hospitals. There are, however, general recommendations issued by the Authority per l'Informatica (Authority for IT) which apply to the whole of the Public Service. A federating element will hopefully be represented by the information requirements that Regional Health Authorities are introducing towards health institutions and health professionals. The need to communicate such information to Health Authorities will standardise the interface of hospital information systems towards the external world and, in parallel, will impose some minimal requirement on the breadth and kind of information that these systems are capable of handling.

A new area of expansion for IT in hospitals is constituted by Executive Information Systems (EIS), as a consequence of the increased control that hospital managers are required to have on the organisations they run[p]. The introduction of IT - especially in respect of EIS - is increasingly considered as a strategic element, since it is capable of supporting the different decision processes at various levels (top management, middle management and professionals) and guiding them towards concrete objectives: cost control and containment; improved efficiency; evaluation and enhancement of service quality.

This evolution on the one hand makes the use of IT an even more important and strategic factor and, on the other hand, highlights the equally important aspect of infrastructures and communication services.

Hospital Information Systems

The market for administrative information systems has been traditionally dominated by solutions running on mainframes, which, although rather outdated, still represent some 40% of the total.

On the other hand, the new generation of solutions, which addresses clinical information and executive information requirements, is based on open systems and is increasingly offered over client-server architectures with graphical user interface.

Until very recently, the leading edge products were designed around industry specific middleware (DHE, SPHERE, REFERENCES), which represented the glue allowing heterogeneous departmental applications to share databases, exchange data and provide services to one another. Olivetti Sanità is the leader in this segment of the market with GESI boasting a few significant references. CAP Gemini, after an attempt to enter the market in the mid-nineties, has wound down its HIS operation in Italy.

---

p   Hospital Managers are no longer part of the civil service and have no guarantee for their jobs if they do not perform

SMS deserves a special mention, because it is the leader for HIS world-wide and because, after a slow start, it is gaining market share in Italy. There are rumours that SMS is considering expanding in Italy through acquisitions. If this is the case, it could rapidly become number one in the country.

In the last few months, new integrated products developed from scratch using the latest development and production environments (MedTrak, OASIS) appear to be gaining ground, especially among private hospitals.

4.8.4   Current status of RHCN

Following the transfer of responsibility for healthcare to Regions, there is no logical justification for a single national healthcare network as is the case in some other countries such as France or the UK.

There is only one real RHCN in operation in Italy, in the Friuli-Venezia-Giulia Region. It is run by INSIEL, a joint venture between FINSIEL and the Regional Government. While the network provides the functionally that a RHCN should offer, the organisation behind it is still hierarchical, and the system architecture is based on obsolete technology (mainframes).

There are plans for RHCNs to be deployed in a few other regions, with Lombardia perhaps leading the group with the SIS (Sistema Informativo Sanitario) initiative. In the context of SIS, a budget of Lit 90 billion has already been approved for the pilot province of Lecco, which should go live in 2000-01.

Beside these major plans, there are a few networks already in place or close to completion, even if none of them is regional in scope. With no attempt to be exhaustive, the following initiatives are known:

- **CUP 2000** is an initiative launched by the City of Bologna and by the City's healthcare providers to offer citizens a comprehensive booking system which allows booking of medical services in any of the healthcare institutions in the city area. The service offering will evolve and will encompass the exchange of laboratory results.

- **Frameworks** is a project carried out in collaboration between Janssen-Cilag and Bull; this consolidates, at ASL level, healthcare information coming from GPs for epidemiological and management purposes.

- **REMEDES** networks in Bergamo and Melegnano (in progress) link GPs and Free Choice Paediatricians to secondary care providers for clinical services (laboratory test request and result reporting, diagnostic procedure request and result reporting, referral, etc.) and booking both interactive and deferred.

None of the initiatives above is directly backed by a Regional Government. This means that there is no commitment to scale up the present trials to embrace the entire region in which the pilot is established.

4.8.5   Industry - companies, products and services for RHCN

In Italy, RHCNs are in their infancy, as was mentioned in the section above. Referring to the examples of networks quoted, the industrial partners behind the current operating networks or trials are:

BULL: The Italian subsidiary of the French group has been collaborating with the pharmaceutical company Janssen-Cilag to develop Frameworks, a comprehensive networking solution which tightly integrates GPs, ASLs and secondary care providers in a network enriched by a wide range of Added Value Services. The system is installed only in Rho, an ASL near Milan, but there are plans to sell the service to other ASLs.

While Frameworks is a very advanced and well thought through service, it has the disadvantage of being tailored to the hierarchical reality of a today's ASL, which controls and which is the point of reference for the healthcare providers in an area. This paradigm could quickly become obsolete if the healthcare market in Italy opens up according to current expectations.

Frameworks was designed initially to satisfy epidemiological requirements, and it shows very sophisticated features in this respect.

FINSIEL: It is the largest outsourcing, consultancy and system integration company in Italy with over 7.000 staff; it is part of the Telecom Italia Group, the ex-monopolistic telecom operator in the country. They are the industrial partner of CUP2000 in Bologna, which is a joint venture between the Bologna City Council, the Bologna Health Authority (AUSL) and the two large Independently Managed Hospitals in the city area, Sant'Orsola-Malpighi and Rizzoli Orthopaedic Institute. Bologna represents today the largest operational healthcare network in Italy, and the oldest one too - it was created in 1990. FINSIEL is promoting the CUP (Centro Unico di Prenotazione – Unified Booking Centre) in other towns, but there is no evidence of other sales for the time being.

FINSIEL is also part of the INSIEL joint venture with Regione Friuli-Venezia Giulia, but INSIEL is not promoting its RHCN expertise outside the boundaries of the region itself, even if specific software products derived from it have been offered by the parent company in other regions.

Olivetti Sanità: This is a medium-size company within the Olivetti Group, totally dedicated to healthcare information solutions. In the last few years it has invested heavily in the development of the REMEDES set of services, co-funded under the TEN-ISDN and the European Telematics Application Programme. REMEDES covers today the whole communication flow between the GP, on one hand, and the other players of the SSN, with the exception, for the time being, of pharmacies. REMEDES, in comparison with Frameworks, is more flexible and can be adapted to practically any kind of health organisation, including liberal medicine systems, but it is lacking the epidemiological feature of the latter.

REMEDES is today in the initial installation phase in the two pilot sites of Bergamo and Melegnano, but a number of commercial negotiations are already underway.

Telecom Italia: There is no known RHCN offering by the largest telecom operator in Italy, except through its subsidiary Finsiel (see above), but the general strategy of the company aims at reducing the reliance on carrier services and at developing a set of sector based value added services. Telecom Italia is likely to play a major role in the deployment of RHCNs in Italy through partnership with both Regional Health Authorities and smaller suppliers with a strong vertical expertise.

4.8.6 Future development of RHCN, 1998 - 2002

RHCNs in Italy will develop in a very patchy way, mirroring the parallel breakdown of the National Health System into Regional Health Systems, which are increasingly bound to grow apart in terms of organisation and health service offerings.

Some regions will launch far-reaching initiatives calling for a large-scale integration of health information across the boundaries of various levels of healthcare, while other regions will fall behind dramatically, with no human or financial resources to develop networks for healthcare.

It the following description, RHCNs will be discussed according to the classification given in section 3.2.3.2:

- metropolitan/regional booking networks;
- integrated regional networks;
- tele-consulting networks;
- other networks.

4.8.6.1 Metropolitan/regional booking networks

This type of network is very popular for the time being, and they enjoy strong political support. However, they have to cope with a few obstacles for their implementation, namely:

- Local Authority and Health Authority boundaries rarely coincide.

- Existing booking systems are different and not interoperable.

- The push for metropolitan booking networks comes mainly from City Authorities, which have no mandate for healthcare.

In spite of these obstacles, projects for metropolitan booking networks flourish because they have a strong impact on the citizens/electors. At the end of 1998, Bologna opened, with a major event, its second generation metropolitan booking network, totally revamped in terms of user interface, accessibility and coverage. Genova has just gone live, and Roma has announced with a great fanfare that the city will implement the largest network of this kind, with the first services operational for the Jubilee of the year 2000.

4.8.6.2 Integrated regional networks

The most advanced of such networks, at least in terms of design, is the SIS (Sistema Informativo Sanitario - Health Information System) of the Lombardia Region, which calls for a pilot site in the Lecco province in the 1999-2000 time frame, for which a substantial budget has been already allocated.

The SIS project is very comprehensive, but it also respects the autonomy of the individual health authorities; these are given freedom of choice in their domain, provided the systems they choose conform to some minimum criteria, especially in terms of export of information towards the upper layers of SIS. The opening of the network to private value added service providers is envisaged, with the normal conditions concerning access to personal medical data; this is strictly restricted to health professionals having the need to know and the consent of the patient.

Other regions might follow suit, possibly through agreements with the Lombardia Region for consultancy or for technology transfer.

There are a few obstacles to consider in the path towards Integrated Regional Networks:

- the ground on which the upper layers of the networks should be built is not necessarily present;
- the complexity of the enterprise is very high;
- the cultural barriers against innovation, control, information sharing, etc.;
- total transparency in healthcare is not in everybody's interest.

In conclusion, smaller regions are likely to wait and see what happens in Lombardia before they commit themselves to such projects.

4.8.6.3 Tele-consulting networks

With the Italian market for healthcare opening up more and more, and with the well-established principle that money follows the patient, there are all the ingredients to mount tele-consulting networks. Examples already exist today, for example Istituto Ortopedico Rizzoli (IOR) of Bologna.

Tele-consulting is today provided to specialists, normally for a second opinion, through agreements between hospitals and Local Health Authorities. As the health system takes on a stronger consumer orientation, an evolution towards a more aggressive use of tele-consulting as a marketing tool to acquire market share should not be ruled out.

Nevertheless, there are still a few obstacles in the way; they stem principally but not exclusively from the lack of clear legal framework for tele-consulting:

- legal liability;
- payments for tele-consulting;
- availability of cheap broad-band connections.

For the reasons mentioned above, tele-consulting networks might well first see the light of day in the private healthcare sector, to serve a customer base of people more concerned about convenience and access to the best expertise around, than about money.

4.8.6.4 Other networks

Other networks will complete the scenario in the 1998-02 time frame:

- Messaging networks.
- Scientific/epidemiological networks.
- Shared care networks.

4.9 Portugal

4.9.1 Healthcare organisation

The country is divided into five Health Regions which are, in turn, sub-divided into sub-regions. For instance, the Health Region of Lisboa and Tejo Valley (population 3.564.800 inhabitants) comprises the sub-regions of Lisboa, Setúbal and Santarém. The sub-region of Lisboa (population 2.351.900 inhabitants) is divided in six health units which aggregate the services provided in the region by primary care (e.g. health centres) and secondary / tertiary care (e.g. hospitals).

The healthcare organisational structure in a region consists of a network of centres with a high degree of heterogeneity from the organisational, logistic and clinical points of view. In Portugal, healthcare services are provided mainly by a National Health System, supported by a ancillary services, private services, and a small number of health insurance schemes. Regarding the delivery of emergency healthcare, the situation is quite similar.

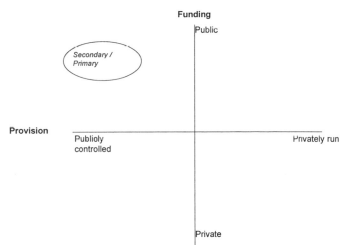

Figure 26: Funding and provision of Portuguese healthcare

A summary of the roles played by the key organisations involved in the healthcare process in the region of Lisboa is shown below:

- ARS (Health Region Administration). ARS is in charge of co-ordinating all the public healthcare organisations within the region, including the definition of healthcare policies, which should be coherent with those derived directly from the Ministry of Health.
- Hospitals provide specialised medical services to citizens. Hospitals are usually classified according to their degree of specialisation and the population they serve, e.g. district, central (university), etc. Hospitals have

their own budget, in part derived from direct billing to healthcare sub-systems, in part funded through the OE (Portuguese Public Budget). Accident and emergency services are mainly provided by hospitals.

- Primary care health centres are the key elements of the healthcare system, and are under the direct administration of ARS. Commonly, a primary care centre serves a population of around 30.000 inhabitants, but occasionally up to 100.000. They are also involved in the accident and emergency process by means of the Serviços de Atendimento Permanente (SAP) (Permanent Attendance Services).

- National Institute for Medical Emergency (INEM) is in charge of the co-ordination of medical emergencies all over the country. In particular, INEM assures the co-ordination of all emergency transport (ambulances), both public and private.

An unquantified number of private clinics, private physicians (general practitioners and specialists), private laboratories, radiology centres, rehabilitation centres, etc., also play a significant role in the provision of care in a region by delivering services either on a private basis, or under some sort of contract to the public system.

4.9.2 Information flows

The typical communication between healthcare providers in a region is summarised in Figure 27 below.

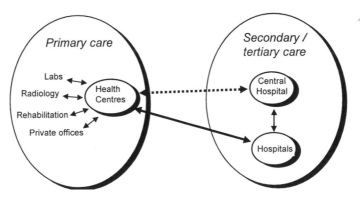

Figure 27: Communications in a region

Communication and data flow between organisations and healthcare professionals are important components of today's healthcare delivery process, and are widely recognised as important causes of wastage of resources and of poor quality of care. The most important communication link is between primary care health centres and hospitals, particularly in the context of health units. Referral of patients from GPs to hospital specialists, together with consequent feedback (e.g. discharge note, or report), are considered the most important information links. A similar but less relevant link exists between hospitals. Another important connection consists of the communication between health professionals, mainly GPs, and the diversity of public and private healthcare providers, of diagnostic and/or treatment procedures (i.e. laboratories, radiology centres, rehabilitation centres, etc.).

4.9.3 IT systems in healthcare

In this last decade, particularly in the last few years, there has been an increasing introduction of information systems in health organisations in Portugal. The first systems introduced in public hospitals only provided administrative functionality, e.g. management of stock and accounting, and have been designed as stand-alone applications or small local networks. Then the Ministry of Health, through the Institute of Informatics and Finances of the Ministry of Health (IGIF), launched a national programme aiming to install in all public hospitals a patient management system called SONHO, developed in-house by IGIF. Several versions of this system have been delivered since then, but again focusing on administrative functionality, including the following modules: patient identification, patient admission / transfer / discharge, outpatients booking / scheduling, and billing.

At the same time, over the last few years IGIF has developed a few other information systems for hospitals such as: DRG (Diagnosis Related Groups) system, pharmacy system, operating theatre information system, and hospital personnel management system. Though a full integration with SONHO has not yet been attained, some communication (e.g. patient identification) between these departmental systems and SONHO is provided.

Initially, SONHO was installed in only a few hospitals, but now there is a programme to generalise its use to all (or most) public hospitals. However, several important hospitals have already acquired other IT solutions, which they will certainly not replace (especially in the case where additional value has been obtained, e.g. better integration).

Concerning the primary care sector, more recently the Ministry of Health launched a similar project aiming to install a patient management system, entitled SINUS, for the primary care health centres; this was also developed in-house by IGIF. Like SONHO, SINUS has been designed mainly for administrative purposes. Some communication between SINUS and SONHO is offered, enabling health centres' users to book directly specialist consultation appointments in the hospital.

In addition to this basic infrastructure, an unknown number of personal databases exist both in primary and secondary care, as well as with private physicians; these are usually used for specialised clinical purposes, e.g. diabetes, hypertension, multiple sclerosis, and many other. Also, a variety of departmental laboratory systems (developed by several sources) exist in public hospitals; most of them are not integrated with the hospital patient management system SONHO.

Finally, a number of application prototypes exist in public healthcare organisations as a direct result of participation in R&D telemedicine / telematic projects, mainly under the European Union IIIrd and IVth Framework Programmes regarding the Healthcare Sector. A few examples of these are: GEHR, Diabcare, Diabcard, Esteem, Hansa, Prestige, Hector, Nivemes, ENN; this list is not exhaustive.

IT providers

Because the provision of healthcare services in Portugal is mostly dependent on a public National Health System (NHS), the present situation regarding the use of IT in healthcare, and of RHCNs in particular, is mainly determined by the state of development in the public sector. Because the Ministry of Health, through IGIF, has been the main IT supplier for the NHS, existing products, services and solutions in most healthcare organisations of the country have been offered by IGIF. This situation has clearly left very little room for industry products / services in a country that already has a small business market.

A few exceptions to such domination by IGIF exist in the public sector. Some hospitals have acquired different hospital information systems from a variety of IT suppliers. In addition, a variety of departmental information systems and specialised applications for clinical purposes also exist in public hospitals and GP centres. The most relevant examples include:

- Laboratory departmental information systems from different IT providers. Most of these systems are adapted to hospitals from solutions developed for private laboratory centres.

- Electronic Medical Record, mainly in the primary care sector.

- A few specialised databases for processing specific datasets / clinical trials regarding well defined medical domains, for example, diabetes, hypertension, epilepsy, etc.

- Some telemedicine applications (i.e. tele-radiology, tele-pathology, remote / home monitoring, etc.), mainly derived from research and development projects, are running in a few hospitals on a prototype basis.

With regard to healthcare sub-systems, insurance systems and the private sector, with the exception of laboratory information systems there is a lack of precise information on the extent, characteristics and sources of existing IT products / solutions.

4.9.4   Current status of RHCN

In 1997, the Ministry of Health, through IGIF, launched a programme aimed at implementing a national information network for health - Rede de Informação na Saúde (RIS) - to connect IGIF regional centres (covering the five Portuguese Health Regions) as well as the health organisations within the Regions. This activity is complemented by another national programme, also launched by IGIF, aimed at implementing a national patient identification number; this will enable the future integration of patient data, bearing in mind the patient management systems developed for primary and secondary care, SINUS and SONHO respectively. Such integration should be achieved, in the first instance, at the health unit / regional level.

Complementing those activities, the Ministry of Health, again through IGIF, launched during 1998 another national programme aimed at generalising the use of an electronic patient card for administrative / management purposes. This electronic patient card is already being utilised, in the primary care sector, in a few Health Regions.

4.9.5 Industry - companies, products and services for RHCN

The state of development of RHCN in Portugal is quite limited. The national information network for health (Rede de Informação da Saúde - RIS) and the communication between SINUS (patient management system for GP centres) and SONHO (patient management system for hospitals) for referral / booking purposes are however already a reality; both of these are implemented by IGIF. The Electronic Patient Card being disseminated by IGIF complements such a strategy through the integration / communication power provided by the national health patient identification number also promoted by IGIF.

Three projects offering solutions for RHCNs, in different stages of development, deserve a few additional comments.

- Regimed Portuguesa: Serviços Médicos S.A. is promoting a solution, entitled 'Solução Vital', aimed at implementing a private health intranet using ISDN. Target users are mainly represented by private physicians. The solution is based on a health card - 'Cartão Vital' - capable of storing clinical and administrative patient data by means of an incorporated microchip. Solução Vital has already come into a commercial phase.

  The most relevant services and functionality provided to users includes:
  - to access, send to and update from a central database the electronic patient card (including images);
  - to produce customised reports, official forms, drug prescriptions, etc.;
  - to perform statistics on the database;
  - to request or send encrypted messages, as well as other patient data including images, via electronic mail from / to other clinicians also using this solution;
  - video-conferencing.

- CENTIS has developed a system for RIICN in the accident and emergency sector. This system entitled EUMed (Sistema de Gestão de Recursos de Emergência e Urgência Médica) aims to provide efficient and easy to use telematic means for optimising the use of the resources provided by healthcare organisations involved in accident and emergency medical care. The system consists of a central database (i.e. regional server) comprising all the information required for processing resources use, together with an application for accessing the central database, as well as a set of telematic services focused on the accident and emergency care sector. Validation of the pilots will start soon.

  EUMed has been in part funded by the European Union under the Telematics Application Programme, Hector Project.

- GeneSys is another solution developed by CENTIS foreseeing the implementation of a RHCN, also by means of ISDN, in a distinct medical area - Clinical Genetics. GeneSys has been primarily designed to support clinical and management activities on a departmental basis. However, the solution offered enables a variety of organisations / clinical departments (i.e. in remote locations) of several medical specialities (i.e. obstetrics, paediatrics, clinical genetics) to share and exchange information for the management of patients and families.

GeneSys is based on a client / server architecture offering to users:
- act management facilities, comprising an explicit monitoring of acts' life-cycle and a requester / performer schema; a typical act life-cycle comprises the following: request, schedule, execute and report;
- a set of facilities for characterising the organisations / actors, particularly to specify who can do what;
- tele-diagnosis;
- video-conferencing.

Validation of the pilots will start soon.

4.9.6 Future development of RHCN, 1998 - 2002

Major developments concerning RHCNs for the period 1998-2002 in Portugal are related to the consolidation of on-going programmes launched by the Ministry of Health described above. The expectations are, first, to install in most hospitals and primary care health centres, the respective patient management systems, either SONHO or SINUS. Then, these health organisations should be progressively integrated into the national health information network RIS. This integration, together with a more general use of the electronic patient card, should enable a proper communication between the variety of healthcare providers at the different levels of the healthcare system. The idea is to enable proper information flow within the different healthcare sectors (e.g. primary care), between sectors (e.g. primary care and secondary care), and between those sectors and management / administration bodies, from the health unit to the regional and national levels.

Finally, the Ministry of Health is starting to consider clinical data as an important element for health information systems. It is expected that an electronic patient record integrated with existing patient management systems will constitute an implementation priority in a near future. Because of the variety and complexity of the electronic patient record, it is also expected that a multiplicity of IT suppliers will develop/adapt IT solutions to the requirements specified by IGIF. The recent announcement from IGIF on putting into the public domain its legacy systems (e.g. SONHO and SINUS) constitutes a clear indicator that a promising new era is starting for the wide dissemination of IT in healthcare. Resource management and quality of care assessment, at the institutional and regional levels (i.e. implementing the concepts of continuity of care and shared / co-operative care), represent additional important domains deserving an emphasis in future healthcare policies. It is imperative for the success of all these actions that a coherent definition of clinical processes and related minimum data be promoted by the Ministry of Health. Actually, this, together with other standardisation actions, should constitute the main focus of IGIF activity in the future.

4.10 Spain

4.10.1 Healthcare organisation

From the beginning of the eighties, the Spanish Sistema Nacional de Salud (National Health System) began to be decentralised, transferring progressively the comprehensive competencies in health to the Autonomous Governments; this process has stopped during the last years, although it will restart. Between 1986 and 1990, the National Health System was made universal, and now takes care of all the population. At present, almost 60% of the population is attended by the Health Services from the regional Governments with competencies in health, and 40% by the National Health Institute (INSALUD) which is responsible to the central Government.

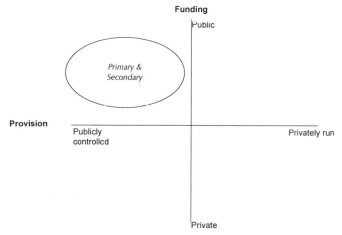

Figure 28: Funding and provision of Spanish healthcare

In the public health sector (with the exception of the military one), all the activity is carried out in health centres classified as Primary Health Care Centres (individual GPs do not exist), Specialists Clinics and Hospitals. All the centres are responsible to either their respective Regional Health Services, or INSALUD through Provincial Head Offices. Exceptionally, the Regional Health Services or the INSALUD have contracts with other private centres (mainly non-profit Institutions); however, in the last years the Central and Autonomous Governments have created their own Foundations by private law - these work for the Health Services on a contract basis. However, for Catalonia this exceptional existence of autonomous Centres is usual. Historically, more than 70% of the hospital activity in Catalonia is carried out, on a contract basis, by several private hospitals (mostly non-profit) and public hospitals (mostly responsible to the City Council). In Catalonia this contractual system is also applied in 10% of primary healthcare.

4.10.2 Information flows

The communication among health centres is mainly by paper. There has been some use of telecommunications in some particular cases; the most advanced regional networks are in the Basque Country, Catalonia and Valencia.

Among the particular cases of electronic communication, we can mention connections between Primary Health Care Centres and hospitals to facilitate the booking of hospital outpatient appointments from Primary Health Care Centres, and some concrete experiences on digital image transmission (CT and MRI).

4.10.3 IT systems in healthcare

Some of these autonomous hospitals were the first ones to introduce Hospital Information Systems (HIS) twenty years ago with Patient Administration System (PAS) models. The PAS implementation was progressive in the eighties, and had a fast expansion at the end of the decade with DIAS Plan. Simultaneously, a lot of hospitals implemented applications for laboratories, in many cases provided by the same suppliers as laboratory material. The progress in the development of the HIS has been quite unequal both in the care aspects (implementation of automated or electronic patient record) and in the economic/ administrative aspects. Nowadays, a few of the 790 Spanish hospitals have already implemented models with a high level of integration in their systems and in the electronic patient record.

There has been lesser implementation of IT in the Primary Health Care Centres. The use of manual booking systems is still the majority overall in Spain, although in some regions they are already totally computerised. It is estimated that GPs with elements of electronic patient record do not reach even 5%.

4.10.4 Current status of RHCN

The network of the Basque Country has been implemented through connections by Euskaltel, the new Basque telecommunications operator. All the health centres and the regional head offices of the Basque Health Service are connected in a voice and data network already used for electronic mail and access to Internet and in the ALDABIDE Project. With this project, already in operation from 1st January 1998, an integrated-decentralised model of economic management has been implemented with software from SAP (purchases, invoicing, accounting, financial management).

The corporate network of the Catalan Health Service has been set up, in a first phase, for the use of the individual health card, for the communication between health centres and users, centres and health institution registries, and for the implementation of patient administration systems in primary health care. It is also used for electronic mail and access to Internet. 290 health centres are connected with one another through 309 lines of data transmission. Within the territory, some 6.000.000 citizens have been identified; of these, 5.000.000 have received a health card that identifies them, assigns them to a Basic Health Area, defines the level of services to which they are entitled, and credits them on the connections points to the network.

The first added value service of the Valencian Health Services network has been the establishment of a Services and Goods Central Purchasing System. 45 management centres (hospitals and Primary Health Care County Head Offices) are connected to a Logistic Central Unit, through a proprietary protocol based on TCP/IP; the Unit is connected to suppliers through EDIFACT.

4.10.5 Industry - companies, products and services for RHCN

The healthcare system decentralisation allied with a prevailing policy of contracting a diversity of HIS suppliers has resulted in different developments and solutions across the regions, with a varying degree of maturity and a large variety of suppliers. Many hospitals have carried out their own developments, home-made or self developed with the support of an SME. Among this diversity, HP (which has announced its withdrawal from the HIS market in many countries but not in Spain), SMS (with more than 50 installations, among them all the military hospitals) and CCS (a Spanish software enterprise which has passed an important crisis) go on standing out.

At the beginning of the nineties, CCS and HP led the hospital software market with approximately 10% each; both are evolving towards a bigger role as implementers and integrators rather than as developers, although HP is offering and installing its more integrated new version HP-HIS-2. Changes are coming about not only in these two enterprises. SMS is starting to implement a new HIS (Aurora) model with GUI and RDBMS developed in Spain; on the other hand, SMS in Andalusia has established a joint venture with an IT company (SADIEL) promoted by the Regional Government. Some hospitals are contracting the Aciva2000 system, an Australian/Spanish development which EDS (USA) and IECISA (one of the Spanish leaders in IS) are betting on. The implementation of this HIS that uses Caché can have an influence on the plentiful installations that work with MUMPS, since not only SMS and CCS use MUMPS, but it is also the main language and database used for the HISs developed by some hospitals themselves. INDRA and INDRA SSI, enterprises of public origin, whose privatisation will be complete in 1998, have inherited and are improving the positions that Eritel, as public enterprise, had in the Spanish hospital market. The Basque hospitals and a University one have adopted the economic/financial integrated system of SAP, which is also offering their German developed care system. Ibermatica, a subsidiary company of IBM, is also increasing its activity. Among the SMEs of regional influence are Valen Computer in Catalonia, SIVSA in Galicia and MBA-Biocon in Asturias. The changes that are being brought about in the HIS market are related to the transition to client-server models and to integrated systems. Within the integrated systems policy, there are some hospitals with home-grown developments, and some enterprises that are implementing the European prestandard of HISA architecture in its DHE version (validated in HANSA, a Project from TAP of EU).

The IS market for primary care centres is mainly distributed among two companies, Stacks and Novasoft, and systems developed by the regional governments. These two companies are also being introduced in the hospital sector.

The only existing application for Nursing houses is Gass developed by CHC and Valen Computer. There are no applications (no home-grown ones) for home care, although the results of the Ithaca Project can be promising.

In applications for Laboratories there are still standing out the ones offered by the laboratory suppliers (Izasa, Bayer, Boehringer, etc.).

There are not too many hospitals working with applications for radiology imaging. In this limited market, initially dominated by suppliers of radiological equipment (Philips, GE, Siemens, etc.), Medasys and E-Med are now developing positions. Siemens, for its part, is commercialising the Raim system developed by the UDIAT public enterprise.

The implementation of EDI in the Spanish health field started exclusively in the hands of TSAI, a subsidiary of Telefonica, until recently a public monopoly. There are already present in the market Fonocom, a subsidiary company of British Telecom, and the Spanish enterprise EDIComunicaciones.

4.10.6 Future development of RHCN, 1998 - 2002

The liberalisation and progress of telecommunications is being translated, initially, by setting up telecommunication regional networks among public buildings, in order to improve their communications and reduce phone costs. These infrastructure policies are important not only in the advanced regions described above, but also in other regions with a lesser use of networks for the health system (for example, in the north-west of Spain: Galicia and Asturias).

Practically, all the regional Governments with competences in health are starting to develop projects of health intranets. Even though some projects are already in the definition phase, described below are the main trends, starting with the initiatives arising in the regions, to evaluate later on the ones that have their origins in projects of the EU.

In Catalonia, the regional health network has as its most immediate objectives
- completion of connection of all the centres;
- finishing the distribution of the individual health cards (the previous health card, already valid in parallel with the new one, did not have magnetic support and it was for a family);
- better use of the information on activity available.

1.850.000 visits to the Primary Health Care Centres are being registered each month, and 99,2 % of the prescriptions are registered once the medicine is delivered to the patient.

Because of the autonomy level of the Catalan health centres, the use of IT for the co-operation and interchange of information depends on their respective decisions. These are being implemented either through centres owned by the same health group, or through ad hoc agreements. Small networks have been set up, in some cases for sharing information of patient records among different healthcare levels, and in other cases to interchange images for sharing radiology images (networks in Emporda, Reus-Tarragona, Terrassa and CHC group). In all these cases with transfer of information, centres use the same applications and proprietary software.

The ALDABIDE Project of the Basque Health Service, initiated in 1996, will be completed at the end of 1998. It is therefore in the consolidation phase, starting the information's exploitation with data contrast (benchmarking), and setting up a personalised information system in all the centres. But this project for economic management is not the only one, neither is it the main objective of the established network. It is expected it will be used for the interchange of information among university hospitals for research, and for transfer of information between primary and specialised healthcare (hospitals included), firstly for booking and later on for patient information. Likewise, the features of the network permit the transfer of diagnostic images. The Basque Health Service policy of contracting the same applications for all the centres, already applied for primary healthcare and for economic management, makes the possibility of information transmission much easier.

The Basque and Catalan Health Services and the Regional Government of Madrid are taking part jointly with the Health Information National Centre (from Instituto de Salud Carlos III) in the care area of PISTA Project from the Telecommunications General Directorate of Ministerio de Fomento. This has as its objectives the development of a data warehouse of clinical information, a common system of activity request management (visits in hospital and primary healthcare and diagnostic tests), as well as a web of general information on health.

The PISTA Project has another health information area that includes all Spain through which there will be connected:
1. units of the Epidemiological Vigilance Network, for statistics, public information and planning through dynamic consultations;
2. the Public Health Laboratories for normalisation and follow up of the information;
3. the regional Agencies of Medical Technology Assessment for sharing public information of the techniques and methods evaluated by the respective Agencies.

The intranet project of the Andalusia Health Service has similar objectives to the PISTA Project.

The Health Department of the Valencian Government counts on several projects for the healthcare use of its network. Besides other projects such as Central Purchases, tele-radiology and teleconferencing, the Abucasis project stands out. Its first phase has already ended. The project implements information systems in Primary Health Care Centres, with possibility of booking by the users from home, through the Internet, and connection with all the specialised care centres for laboratory requests and results.

From the EU Telematic Applications Programme, we should mention the CoCo, CHIN, HECTOR and REMEDES projects; they are all promising projects, implementing results in Spanish RHCNs.

In the CoCo Project, EDIFACT messages between hospital and primary healthcare are being implemented and validated in Barcelona and Palma de Mallorca. During the project, centres of the two levels from the Manacor (Mallorca) area have already been added and centres from other areas of Catalonia, Aragon and Andalusia have expressed their interest in applying the model.

Since the end of 1997, the Health Resources Directory of the Catalan Health Service, in the health region of Costa de Ponent (1,1 million inhabitants) is available on Internet. It has been developed on the basis of the methodology of the CHIN Project, with more than 600 web pages of information about more than 200 health centres. It is expected that the CHIN model of the Resources Directory will be spread to other regions. Some health centres are also using the CHIN guidelines to develop their own webs.

The technologies developed within the HECTOR project in Andalusia with use of telematics for medical emergencies is being evaluated in other regions for its use.

4.11   UK

4.11.1 Healthcare organisation

The UK operates a public healthcare system, the National Health System (NHS), funded through national taxation. Healthcare in England and Wales is managed by the NHS Executive (NHSE) reporting to the Department of Health, while healthcare in Scotland and Northern Ireland is managed by the Scottish Office and Northern Ireland Office respectively.

The organisation of the NHS in Wales, Scotland and Northern Ireland is broadly similar to that in England, although there are differences in naming the various components. Within England there are eight Regions. Wales, Scotland and Northern Ireland can each be considered as regions. Described below is the organisation of the NHS for England.

The principal actors within the English health service, and a summary of their responsibilities, are:

- NHS Executive: This is the top management tier of the NHS. It is part of the Department of Health, and is responsible to Ministers; it has overall responsibility for provision of healthcare, and sets strategic direction in a number of areas.

- Regions: There are eight Regional Offices; these are responsible for setting direction, targets and budgets within their areas, and monitoring performance. The Regional Offices report to the Executive.

- Health Authorities (HAs): These are responsible primarily for directing and monitoring healthcare provision, both primary and secondary. HAs report to Regions.

- General Practitioners (GPs): These provide primary healthcare to patients. GPs are self-employed independent contractors.

- Hospitals and Community Trusts: These provide secondary (and in some cases tertiary) healthcare to patients. Although these are directly part of NHS, they have considerable autonomy to manage their affairs, and report to Regional Offices.

- Social Services Departments of local Councils: responsible for non-medical care of the elderly and mentally ill within the community environment.

Within the NHS, health provision is organised along "Purchaser" and "Provider" lines. Purchasers are responsible for determining the health needs of their local population, and allocating the funds for healthcare appropriately. Healthcare provision is then "purchased" from Providers, who are responsible for delivering the healthcare services required; in general, Providers deliver one or more of specific types of healthcare, e.g. hospital services, or community services.

Within the NHS, purchasing is carried out by HAs and Primary Care Groups, a new level of purchaser organisation which is taking over responsibility for purchasing healthcare on behalf of all GPs in the Group; these were introduced in April 1999. Through private healthcare insurance, insurance companies such as BUPA and PPP can also be considered as Purchasers.

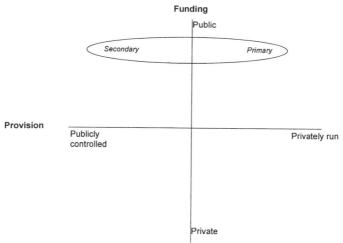

Figure 29: Funding and provision of UK healthcare

Providers within the NHS comprise GPs, acute and community Trusts, dentists, and similar health professionals.

The numbers of regions, Health Authorities and Trusts in England, Wales, Scotland and Northern Ireland are shown in Table 14 below.

Table 14: Health Authorities and Trusts in UK

Regions	HAs	Trusts
England		
• Anglia & Oxford Region	9	45
• North Thames Region	14	62
• North West Region	16	61
• Northern & Yorkshire Region	13	52
• South & West Region	12	48
• South Thames Region	12	63
• Trent Region	11	43
• West Midlands Region	13	50
Total for England	100	424
Northern Ireland	4	20
Scotland	15	47
Wales	5	29

The total spending on the NHS for 1997/98 year was some 62 billion euros, while the spending on private healthcare is estimated at 11 billion euros. Within the UK, England accounts for approximately 75% of the healthcare expenditure.

4.11.2 Information flows

There are two principal categories of information flow:
- flows to support the clinical treatment of patients; these are as described at the start of this section;
- administrative flows to support the contracting (and management) arrangements.

The diagram below shows the main administrative flows. With the introduction of Primary Care Groups in 1999, there is likely to be some change to the flow of contracting data.

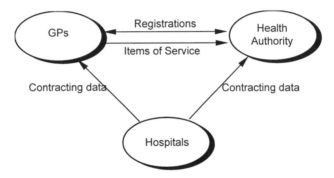

Figure 30: Administrative information flows in UK

4.11.3 IT systems in healthcare

Primary Care

Within the UK, over 90% of GP practices have some form of computer system installed, with over 50% of these systems providing clinical records.

Primary Care Systems

While in 1993 there were 104 suppliers providing specialist GP computer software[20], this number has reduced dramatically, particularly with the introduction of the NHSE's Requirements for Accreditation programme. In 1995 there were 18 suppliers of accredited systems. The market in England and Wales is now dominated by three suppliers: Reuters Health (formerly VAMP), EMIS, and AAH Meditel, while in Scotland GPASS Unit is also a major supplier.

Secondary Care

Within the secondary care sector, virtually all hospitals have IT systems in support of clinical activities, though the take up of such systems in different areas varies. The areas where IT systems are most common are:
- patient administration systems (PAS);

- outpatient booking;
- waiting list management;
- pharmacy;
- laboratory systems (pathology, etc.).

The NHS Executive has a well defined Information Management & Technology strategy. The key features are:

- person based information;
- integrated systems;
- management information derived from operational systems and data;
- secure and confidential information;
- shared information across the NHS;
- new (unique) NHS number.

In addition, IT systems for administrative support are normal; these are often standard, commercially available packages, albeit adapted where necessary to specific NHS requirements:

- accounting systems
- personnel
- payroll.

While many of the existing clinical and administrative systems installed at the moment may need to be replaced/upgraded to meet changing business needs or to make use of new technologies, in general much of the routine operation of hospitals is now supported by IT systems; further progress in these areas will be evolutionary, rather than revolutionary.

However, increasingly, IT systems are being introduced in such areas as Executive Information Systems (EIS), decision support, and expert systems. These systems could have dramatic effects on the value that hospitals can get from the existing data. Because these are new areas, there is much less commonality in approach.

Secondary Care Systems

In secondary care, there are three suppliers with a major share of the market for hospital systems: HBOC, Siemens Nixdorf, and SMS. However, there are at least another 10 suppliers in this market.

Other secondary care systems that are relevant for RHCNs include radiology and pathology systems.

4.11.4 Current status of RHCN

Since 1995, the NHS Executive in England has been implementing an NHS wide network, NHSnet. NHSnet comprises a national spine network, linking various regional networks, and is a key element of the Information Management and Technology strategy for the NHS; there is also a connection to the Racal Healthlink network - this predates NHSnet, and is a messaging network linking GPs and Health Authorities. The aim of NHSnet is to enable all parts of the NHS to communicate with each other efficiently, securely, and cost-effectively, exploiting modern communications technologies. NHSnet:

- allows GPs to communicate with HAs, acute and community Trusts and other organisations throughout the NHS;

- provides all NHS organisations with connections to national bodies including NHS Supplies, NHS Central Register, the Dental Practice Board, and the Prescription Pricing Authority;

- allows providers and purchasers to exchange contracting data;

- provide secure links to organisations outside the NHS, for example to suppliers using EDI, and Internet.

A number of national applications are offered over NHSnet. These include:

- The NHS Managed Message Handling Service (MMHS). This provides an X.400 based message handling service, and X.500 directory service. MMHS links with Racal's Healthlink service.

- The NHS-Wide Clearing Service (NWCS). This provides a service for the delivery of the Contract Minimum Data Sets (CMDSs) which flow between providers and purchasers to allow the internal NHS market to function.

- The NHS Strategic Tracing Service (NSTS). This will provide a service to trace users of the NHS to ensure the correct unique NHS number is used.

In addition to these national applications, NHSnet is being used for general health service business. Of relevance to RCHNs are the following:

- The GP Provider Links project has been set up by the NHS Executive to pilot national EDIFACT standards for test results, discharge summaries, etc. These pilots are using NHSnet to connect hospitals and GPs.

- NHSnet is also aimed at carrying "content only" information services, either through Web sites connected directly to NHSnet, or by providing a secure gateway to such services carried on the Internet. This is generically referred to as NHSweb.

4.11.5 Industry - companies, products and services for RHCN

Within the UK, there are two principle providers of networks for RHCNs, British Telecom (BT) and Cable & Wireless (formerly Mercury). These two companies have won framework contracts for the supply of regional networks, while BT has the contract for the "spine" network to connect RHCNs into NHSnet. In addition, Racal operates Healthlink, the messaging network linking GPs to Health Authorities for the exchange of Registration and Items of Service information.

In addition to the basic network provision, BT Syntegra operates the X.400 Managed Message Handling Service (MMHS), and an X.500 directory service. The contract for the NHS-Wide Clearing Service (NWCS) was won by AT&T, now taken over by HBOC.

With regard to companies supplying healthcare application products to the primary and secondary care markets, there has been a significant shakeout in the market over the last few years, with suppliers selling their healthcare divisions to other companies.

All suppliers of application systems are under pressure to exchange patient healthcare information electronically, for example results reporting and discharge summaries. This process has been given significant impetus through the GP Links project, which is setting EDIFACT standards.

4.11.6 Future development of RHCN, 1998 - 2002

As has been described above, the UK already has a national healthcare network in place, NHSnet.

Most health authorities and secondary care providers are linked to this network, but very few GPs. However, the government has put in place a programme (GPnet) to connect all GPs/GP practices to NHSnet by the end of 1999. In conjunction with this, GP system suppliers have been targeted with upgrading their systems so that they can receive pathology results conforming to the EDIFACT National Standard Message (NSM) via NHSnet.

This means that by the year 2000, virtually all healthcare organisation will be connected to the national NHSnet healthcare network.

Following on from this, the NHS can be expected to increase the number of mandated clinical messages. These are already being trialled through the GP Provider Links project. In addition, the government wishes to see GPs making outpatient bookings by the end of year 2001.

Also as a result of this, Web based services can be expected to increase, although here the NHS is more likely to let market forces set the pace.

A key issue still to be resolved in achieving these targets is establishing an acceptable security (encryption) regime to ensure clinical data is never in the clear outside of the relevant clinical domains. In this context, acceptable means effective, and affordable.

Appendix A

Glossary and Abbreviations

AIM	Advanced Informatics in Medicine; part of European Union IIIrd Framework Programme
ANSI	American National Standards Institute
API	Application Programme Interface
ARS	In Portugal, the Regional health authority
ASL	In Italy, Aziende Sanitarie Locali (Local Health Authority)
ATM	A telecommunication network protocol
Aziende Ospedaliere	In Italy, Independently Managed Hospital
Azicnde Sanitaric Locali	In Italy, Local Health Authority, replacing Unità Sanitarie Locali (q.v.)
BPR	Business Process Re-engineering
CEN	Committee European de Normalisation, or European Standardisation Committee
CME	Continuing Medical Education; and alternative term for CPD (q.v.)
CNIL	In France, Commission Nationale de l'Informatique et des Libertés
CPD	Continuing Professional Development
CT	Computer Tomography
DRG	Diagnosis Related Group
EAN	European Article Numbering; scheme which assigns unique number to every supplier, and hence every article or goods that can be ordered.
EBES	European Board for EDI Standardisation
ECG	Electrocardiogram
ECR	Electronic (Health) Care Record
EDI	Electronic Data Interchange
EDIFACT	
EFTA	European Free Trade Area

EIS	Executive Information System; term used in IT to refer to software tool to manipulate data for management queries and reporting.
EHCR	Electronic Health Care Record; often used synonymously with EPR (q.v.)
EPR	Electronic Patient Record; often used synonymously with EHCR (q.v.)
GDP	Gross Domestic Product
GNP	Gross National Product
GP	General Practitioner; although not all countries have GPs, the term is used generically to refer to doctors practising in primary care
GSM	Global Satellite Monitoring
Health Board	In Ireland, the regional health authority In Scotland and Northern Ireland, the local health authority
HIS	Hospital Information System, or Health Information System
HISA	Health Information System Architecture
HL7	Protocol for exchanging (electronic) messages containing health information
HTML	Hyper Text Mark-up Language
ICD	International Classification of Diseases
ICPC	International Classification for Primary Care
ICT	Information and communication technology
IGIF	In Portugal, the Institute of Informatics and Finances, within the Ministry of Health
IMH	Independently Managed Hospitals
IM&T	Information Management and Telecommunications
INEM	In Portugal, National Institute for Medical Emergencies
INSALUD	In Spain, the National Health Institute, responsible to central Government

ISDN	Integrated Switched Digital Network; a telecommunication network protocol
ISO	International Standards Organisation
ISP	Internet Service Provider, or Integrated Service Provider
ISSS	Information Society Standardisation System
IST	The EU Information Society Technologies programme
IT	Information Technology
Kassenärztliche Vereinigungen	In Germany, regional organisation responsible for reimbursing primary care costs
KV	In Germany, Kassenärztliche Vereinigungen (q.v.)
LAN	Local Area Network
LHA	Local Health Authority, a generic term used within the report; Local Health Authorities typically work within the framework of a Regional Health Authority
MRI	Magnetic Resonance Imaging
NHS	National Health System
NMR	Nuclear Magnetic Resonance
OPCS	In UK, Office for Population Census and Statistics, now replaced by Office of National Statistics (ONS). OPCS-4 is a coding system for operative procedures.
OSI	Open System Interconnection; often refers to seven layer model for systems connection
PC	Personal Computer
Requirements for Accreditation	In UK, programme for defining standard required facilities in GP systems; meeting these requirements is a pre-requisite for reimbursement of costs.
R&D	Research & Development
RfA	In UK, Requirements for Accreditation programme (q.v.)
RHCN	Regional Health Care Network
RIS	In Portugal, Health Information Network

RSS   In France, Réseau Santé Social, a national network for healthcare and social services

SAP   In Portugal, Permanent Attendance Service

SCSSI   In France, Service Central de la Sécurité des Systèmes d'Information

SGML   Standard Generalised Mark-up Language

SIS   In Italy, Health Information System

SME   Small or medium sized enterprise

SNOMED   Systematic Nomenclature for Medicine and Veterinary Science; a pathology based coding system originating in USA.

SSN   Italian National Health System

TAP   European Union, Telematics Application Programme

TCP/IP   Transfer Control Protocol / Internet Protocol

Unità Sanitarie Locali   In Italy, Local Health Unit, being replaced by Aziende Sanitarie Locali (q.v.)

USL   In Italy, Unità Sanitarie Locali (Local Health Unit)

VANS   Value Added Network Service; refers to services offered over telecommunication networks, over and above the basic communication service.

WWW or www   World Wide Web

XML   Extended Mark-up Language

Appendix B

Healthcare Standardisation Organisations

B.1   Status of the standardisation organisations: CEN TC251

It was only with the introduction of telematics in healthcare that an urgent need was revealed for organised standardisation activities, and for a common use of standards in healthcare informatics, in particular basic standards securing compatibility, connectivity and interchangeability. In order to respond to this challenge, the Technical Board of the European Standardisation Committee (CEN/BT) approved the establishment of a Technical Committee for Medical Informatics (TC 251) in March 1990.

Since any standardisation activity should begin by identifying the needs and determining the aims of the (pre)-standard(s) to be prepared and the interests that may be affected, CEN issued a mandate (BC-IT-SI-05) to assess the current situation of standardisation in Medical Informatics.

The recommendations originating from this mandate are part of CEN/TC 251's "Directory of the European Standardisation Requirements and Programme for the Development of Standards for Healthcare Informatics" in which the tasks for the Working Groups (WGs) and Project Teams (PTs) are described.

The major goal of this committee is to develop standards for communication among independent medical information systems so that clinical and management data produced by one computer system could be transmitted to another system (e.g. the computer system in the ordering physician's practice). Such standards could lead to many improvements and efficiencies in clinical care, research and administration.

CEN/TC 251 establishes priorities based on healthcare market priorities and identifies both publicly available specifications (PAS) and outputs from R&D programmes (e.g. AIM, Advanced Informatics in Medicine / Health Telematics, DG XIII-C4) which are suitable for rapid transformation into standards.

When the market is not providing the solutions, CEN/TC 251 generates suitable standards through consensus-building. The major objectives of CEN/TC 251 are reflected in its structure of Working Groups and in its Project-Teams' activities.

The original seven Working Groups in CEN/TC 251 were:
WG 1:   Healthcare Information Modelling and Medical Records
WG 2:   Healthcare Terminology, Semantics and Knowledge Bases
WG 3:   Healthcare Communications and Messages
WG 4:   Medical Imaging and Multimedia
WG 5:   Medical Device Communication in Integrated Healthcare
WG 6:   Healthcare Security and Privacy, Quality and Safety
WG 7:   Intermittently Connected Devices (including Cards)

In 1997, the scope of TC251 was slightly modified from Medical informatics into Health informatics. At the same time, the seven working groups were reorganised into four new ones:
WG I: Information Models
WG II: Terminology
WG III: Security, Safety and Quality

WG IV: Technology for Interoperability

The objectives of CEN/TC 251 are the organisation, the co-ordination and the follow-up of standards' development in Healthcare Informatics and Telematics, at a European level (15 EU countries, three EFTA countries and a growing number of Eastern European countries).

CEN/TC 251 has so far been a successful Technical Committee. It has produced a number of pre-standards (ENVs) and CEN Reports (CRs) (technical reports). About 1500 experts (from 30 different countries) participate in the efforts, either on a voluntary basis (in Delegations at the Committee level, in Working Groups and in National Mirror Groups) or mandated by the Commission of the European Union (in Project Teams).

The importance of the CEN standards is the agreement of its member countries to accept the CEN standards (not pre-standards) as national standards.

WG I, Information Models

Healthcare is an information-intensive and a communications-intensive business. The volume of information exchanged between departments within hospitals and between primary and secondary care providers is large. Some 15% of a hospital's running costs and 25% of the time of doctors and nurses are devoted to information processing[21].

Electronic data interchange (EDI) offers large potential benefits within healthcare. EDI guarantees the connection and offers security and reliability. Patients benefit as a result of reduced delays and improved availability of information, resulting in quicker and more soundly based clinical decisions. Productivity is improved by reducing the time spent waiting for, or looking for, information and re-entering data into computers, thereby reducing the costs of care.

The scope of WG I is the development of European standards to facilitate communication between independent information systems within and between organisations, for health related purposes.

Such standards are essential if healthcare services are to obtain the benefits of open systems and avoid the constraints of proprietary interfaces. The standards are based on information models - generic models of aspects of health care or health care information. WG I will therefore develop domain model based reference architectures for evolutionary information systems. These will facilitate optimised health care processes for maximum patient perceived quality satisfaction, workflow oriented polycentric care and approaches to archiving healthcare information, that are not time limited

An important area of WG I work is standards for the Electronic Healthcare Record. These will include a record architecture establishing the principles for representing the information content and record structure, a set of concepts and terms for record components, and rules and mechanisms for sharing and exchanging records. A domain model representing a formal description of the context, within which the healthcare records are used, will be established to document requirements for these standards.

Another important area of WG I work is that of standards for messages to meet specific healthcare business needs for the communication of healthcare information. While some messages may have a broad initial scope, WG I will also validate, refine and profile these and other messages to ensure they are applicable to specialist domains with particular requirements. WG I will also address the maintenance, revision and harmonisation of existing message standards.

The standards developed by WG I should enable the information that supports patient care to be communicated unambiguously in order to enhance the quality of care. Therefore, WG I will liaise with WG II to ensure that terminology standards are taken into account and appropriately utilised in standards for healthcare communication.

WG II, Terminology

The objectives of CEN/TC 251 WG II are the semantic organisation of information and knowledge so as to make it of practical use in the domains of health informatics and telematics, and the provision of information and criteria to support harmonisation. This encompasses clinical, managerial and operational aspects of the medical record, and enabling access to other knowledge.

The actual work items focus on:
- terms, concepts and the interrelationship of concepts;
- structures for concepts systems, including those for multi-axial coding schemes;
- guidelines for the production of coding systems and knowledge bases.

Production of coding systems is outside the scope of the Working Group.

WG III, Security, Safety and Quality

The current European and national legislation emphasises the importance of quality, safety and security. It provides a statutory framework to ensure that information systems used in healthcare have appropriate levels of quality, safety and security. Major pan-European documents that provide a basis for CEN/TC 251 are the recommendations from the Council of Europe which apply to all CEN nations, and the European Union Data Protection Directive finally adopted in 1995, to be implemented in member states by October 1998.

It must be emphasised that standards for security, safety and quality must be developed in parallel with the basic informatics standards, for example healthcare communication or electronic record systems. Without considering these important regulatory aspects, the technical possibilities for important efficiency improvements using health telematics cannot be fully exploited.

- **Security** of information systems is usually defined as the prevention of breaches of confidentiality, integrity and availability. In healthcare information systems, the main reason for the major concern with confidentiality is the protection of the privacy of the individual. Patients have to trust healthcare establishments to look after for the very sensitive information they give them. In this context, systems have to be understood in a wider sense, including the surrounding procedures.

- **Safety** of systems can be defined as the expectation that systems do not, under defined conditions, enter a state that could cause human death or injury. In this definition, however, a 'system' will include the software, the hardware, the users of the system and the procedures and practices related to the working of the system. It is not sufficient to analyse a software system without considering how it is used and the environment in which it is used. Software does not actually kill or injure people - it is the associated hardware or the actions of inaccurately informed staff that may cause harm.

- **Quality** is defined as: the totality of features and characteristics of a product, process or service that bear on its ability to satisfy its stated or intended needs. Two important features of the overall quality of such systems are the safety and the security of the systems, and these elements will become even more important as information systems are increasingly used for safety- and security-critical applications.

It is expected that future development of IT security will take place in the following arenas:
- development of protection profiles for various sectors or application areas;
- development of detailed protocols for various core security services;
- evaluation and certification of IT products;
- evaluation, certification and accreditation of IT systems.

Of course, care should be taken to include ethical and juridical notions in these considerations. Although no clear framework exists for this, it could be said that WG III should 'audit' other work within the sphere of CEN/TC 251. The WG could identify and give advice on all relevant security, safety and quality related issues and ensure that issues of a general nature are developed as application independent standards in WG III to achieve consistency.

WG IV, Technology for Interoperability

The aim of WG IV is to develop and promote standards that enable the interoperability of devices and information systems in health informatics.

The scope covers three main areas:
- intercommunication of data between devices and information systems;
- integration of data for multimedia representation;
- communication of such data between source departments and other legitimate users elsewhere in the healthcare sector, in order to facilitate electronic healthcare record provision.

The main concern of the WG is technology for interoperability. In addressing this, the issues of methodology, quality, security and architecture will require liaison with the other WGs, other standards bodies and integration activities.

Devices include, for example: clinical analysers, medical imaging and Intensive Care Unit equipment, clinical workstations and cards.

B.2   Status of the standardisation organisations: ISO TC215 for Health Informatics

CEN believes that some of the issues related to such standardisation require co-operation and harmonisation among world-wide efforts, including the initiatives in the United States. In order for CEN/TC 251 to obtain a unified USA response to its proposals, and to establish liaison with USA standards efforts, the Secretary-General of CEN asked ANSI to play a co-ordinating role for the different USA standards efforts.

The ISO technical committee number 215 was established in 1998 as a world-wide standardisation group.

The proposed scope of this group is Standardisation in the field of information for health, and health Information and Communications Technology (ICT) to achieve compatibility and interoperability between independent systems. Also, to ensure compatibility of data for comparative statistical purposes (e.g., classifications), and to reduce duplication of effort and redundancies.

It is not the intent of the ISO/TC215 scope to:
- standardise the clinical practice of medicine;
- define a standardised healthcare delivery service structure;
- standardise medical knowledge, although the representation and exchange of knowledge is within the scope of ISO/TC 215;
- standardise the performance of healthcare, although the definition of standardised comparative performance data is within the scope of ISO/TC215;
- standardise the internal operation of systems and devices, although the standardisation of data structure and the data output from systems and devices is within the scope of ISO/TC215.

The following working groups are proposed:
Working Group 1 – Health Records and Modelling Co-ordination
Working Group 2 - Messaging and Communication
Working Group 3 – Health Concept Representation
Working Group 4 – Security

The scope of effort of the Working Group on Messaging and Communications is defined in three sections.
- Clinical messaging. Advance standards for data interchanges within and between health services entities that support the delivery and management of healthcare and wellness services to an international population.

- Medical device communication. Advance standards for data interchange between medical devices and instruments and between those devices and other health information systems to support the exchange of health related data.

- Business and financial messaging. Advance standards for data interchange within and between health services entities and between those entities and their financial or business partners, including sponsoring authorities, clients, consumers and subjects of care.

B.3   Status of the standardisation organisations: UN/EDIFACT

Overview

The EDIFACT standard ISO 9735 is currently the preferred syntax for implementation of EDI messages within administration, trade and also healthcare in Europe. This syntax is also the one selected by the CoCo project for widespread implementation.

The EDIFACT syntax is maintained by the UN/CEFACT organisation. UN/CEFACT is the United Nations Centre for Facilitation of Procedures and Practices for Administration, Commerce and Transport. It is open to participation from UN member states, intergovernmental organisations and sectorial and industry associations recognised by the Economic and Social Council of the United Nations (ECOSOC). The Centre's objective is to be "inclusive", and it actively encourages organisations to contribute and help develop its recommendations and standards.

The participation of many private-sector associations in UN/CEFACT's work at the policy level, and of hundreds of private-sector technical experts in UN/CEFACT working groups, is a unique feature of the Centre, which is forging new co-operative relationships between private business and public organisations.

Within the United Nations, UN/CEFACT is located in the Economic Commission for Europe (UN/ECE), which is part of the United Nations network of regional commissions. These regional commissions report to the highest United Nations body in the area of economics, trade and development: ECOSOC.

The mission is to improve the ability of business, trade and administrative organisations, from developed, developing and transitional economies, to exchange products and relevant services effectively - and so contribute to the growth of global commerce

EBES - European Board for EDI Standardisation

The representation of UN/EDIFACT in Western Europe was formerly handled by Western Europe EDIFACT Board (WEEB) but is now handled by EBES. This is a structure set up by CEN in conjunction with the communities of economic and governmental interests concerned with the development of EDI standardisation at National and European levels, and with the participation of CENELEC and ETSI. EBES aims at facilitating in Western Europe the development, maintenance and use of UN/EDIFACT standards and of EDI in general, in accordance with international developments, as well as to serve as a forum for the co-ordination of standardisation in the field of data interchange in its broadest sense.

The organisation of EBES has been repeatedly modified. For the moment EBES is a part of the European ISSS initiative. organised as a workshop with a secretariat.

EEG09 - Healthcare messages

The aim of the group is to develop UN/EDIFACT messages in healthcare. The group will manage the process of harmonising healthcare interchange structures of medical, person related, administrative and financial information with the UN/EDIFACT process to secure the availability of UN/EDIFACT messages to meet the requirements of the healthcare community.

The group works closely with CEN TC251 Health Informatics, especially WG I Information Models, on message development. No message under joint development will be sent forward for final approval without their agreement. The group will recognise the role of the CEN TC in managing the process of securing consensus on message functions and their content for healthcare interchanges.

The group also works closely with the Pan-European User group EMEDI to promote the use of UN/EDIFACT in healthcare and administration.

B.4   Status of the standardisation organisations: Some notes about HL7

HL7 was founded in 1987 in USA to develop standards for the electronic interchange of clinical financial and administrative information among independent healthcare oriented computer systems, e.g. hospital information systems, clinical laboratory systems, enterprise systems and pharmacy systems.

The term "Level 7" refers to the highest level of the Open System Interconnection (OSI) model of the International Standards Organisation (ISO). This is not to say that HL7 conforms specifically to ISO defined elements of the OSI's seventh level. Also, HL7 does not specify a set of ISO approved specifications to occupy layers 1 to 6 under HL7's abstract message specifications. HL7 does, however, conform to the conceptual definition of an application-to-application interface placed in the seventh layer of the OSI model.

In the OSI conceptual model, the functions of both communications software and hardware are separated into seven layers, or levels. The HL7 standard is primarily focused on the issues that occur within the seventh, or application level. These are the definitions of the data to be exchanged, the timing of the exchanges, and the communication of certain application specific errors between the applications.

However, of necessity, protocols that refer to the lower layers of the OSI model are sometimes mentioned to help implementers understand the context of the standard. They are also sometimes specified to assist implementers in establishing working HL7-based systems.

The HL7 Working Group is composed of volunteers who give their time on a personal basis or under sponsorship of their employers. Membership in the HL7 Working Group has been, and continues to be, open to anyone wishing to contribute to the development and refinement of Level 7 Interface Standard for network technology in healthcare.

In the last four years its membership has tripled to over 4,400 hospital, professional society, healthcare industry, and individual members, including almost all of the major healthcare systems consultants and vendors. The HL7 standard is supported by most system vendors and used in the majority of large US hospitals today. It is also used in Australia, Austria, Germany, Holland, Israel, Japan, New Zealand and the United Kingdom.

In June of 1994, HL7 was designated by the American National Standards Institute (ANSI) as an ANSI accredited standards developer. The consensus standard was balloted under ANSI rules. HL7 submits this standard to ANSI for consideration as an American National Standard.

The current standard defines transactions for transmitting data about patient registration, admission, discharge and transfers, insurance, charges and payers, orders and results for laboratory tests, image studies, nursing and physician observations, diet orders, pharmacy orders, supply orders, and master files. HL7 is currently developing transactions for exchanging information about appointment scheduling, problem lists, clinical trial enrolments, patient permissions, voice dictation, advanced directives, and physiologic signals. Task forces in HL7 are also busy developing prototype transactions with new state-of-the-art technologies.

B.5 XLM as a syntax for EDI messaging

XML (Extended Mark-up Language) was first conceived in 1996 and became a standard in February 1998. It has been adopted by both Microsoft and Netscape.

It is closely based on SGML (Standard Generalised Mark-up Language), an international standard for the definition of device independent, system independent methods of representing text in electronic form in the same way as HTML. Strictly speaking, SGML is a meta-language for formally describing a mark-up language.

The success of the web is built on three key ideas:
- the Internet and TCP/IP communication protocols;
- hypertext links to multimedia documents;
- mark-up language HTML, a standardised format which work with most workstations enabling the reader to work with a document irrespective of how it was originally prepared (it only specifies how information is to be displayed, it does not describe what it is).

The cross platform independence of the web means that information (including images and other multimedia components) can be viewed on whatever equipment is available.

The Internet provides authorised users with access to any document wherever they are. This means that hospital consultants can easily review patient information at night from their home or while at a conference overseas provided access to this information is allowed. On the other hand, the technology is inexpensive and widely available.

HTML provides good tools for viewing text documents and images, and limited facilities for data collection using text boxes, check boxes and radio buttons, reset and submit buttons.

However, HTML focuses mainly on the display format of information. It is designed to allow documents to be browsed and printed on a wide range of platforms. Thus it supports application to person communication, not EDI.

The new XML technology does not do away with the need to agree standards or for translation. These tasks have to be performed. But now, by using XML the information exchanges can be much more flexible in structure. Also, XML content handling is currently being built-in directly to both web and desktop software suites.

XML will allow data to be exchanged, regardless of the computing systems or accounting applications being used. XML provides the means to separate the data and structure in electronic business documents from the processes. Finally, it promises to make EDI economic and attractive for a mass market.

The use of XML as message syntax does not require any fundamental changes to the communicating clinical applications. The only differences are in the manner in which messages are translated by the EDI interfaces.

In order to have common XML-tags used in different applications, a large task of standardising concepts has to be performed. Again, this will be able to reuse the experiences gained by implementing traditional EDI messages using EDIFACT, HL7, etc.

The Internet technology will allow a large number of different techniques to be used, more or less wiping out the difference between EDI and e-mail. Typically, we will not only have transfer of structured information between applications as in EDI, or transfer of unstructured information between persons as in e-mail, but also we will have all sorts of mixture of structured and unstructured information to also be exchanged between applications and persons.

Currently the implementations in this area are pilots demonstrating the various functionality, but a big effort is needed to standardise the useful combinations and to focus on a small number of useful techniques.

Appendix C

References

[1]   The Missing Link – The Regional Health Care Data Network. EU/AIM. 1994.

[2]   IT-communication in the County of Funen. County of Funen. 1991.

      IT crossing borders. Danish Hospital Institute. 1991.

      KASIK – Mapping internal hospital communication. Kommunedata, Fyns Amt og Bisballe Planlægning. 1992.

      Network in the Odder-region. Fischer og Lorenz/Århus Amt. 1993.

      The Missing Link. The regional health care data network. EU AIM office/Fyns Amt 1994.

      Strategies for Telematics in Metropolitan Areas to Improve Health Care Delivery. EU-AIM office/Anderson Consulting. 1993.

      The Funen Health Care Data Network FynCom. Danish Hospital Institute. 1995.

      Telematics in Primary Care in Europe. IOS Press volume 20. 1995.

      PrimSIFT: An Investigation into the future of Telematics in Primary and Community Care. IOS Press volume 24. 1995.

      EDI forHealth- State of the Art in European Healthcare EDI. EU/EMEDI. 1995.

      Computer-based Shared Care. Erasmus University of Rotterdam. 1995.

      Trends in Health Telematics in the European Union. David Preston, NHS-IMG. 1996.

      TELMED - The Impact of Telematics on the Healthcare. EU/Health Telematics. 1997.

[3]   Kasik – Kortlægning af sygehusenes interne kommunikation. Kommunedata, Fyns Amt og Bisballe Planlægning. 1992.

[4]   FynCom – det fynske sundhedsdatanet. Danish Hospital Institute. 1995.

[5]   Computer-based Shared Care – a study of EDI Applied to Diabetes Care. Peter Branger. 1995.

[6]   Survey of internal communication in Danish Hospitals. Kommunedata I/S, Jens Bisballe Planlaegning A/S. 1992

[7]   Evaluation of a regional electronic health care network – consequences for general practice. Torben Jorgensen and Bent Danneskiold-Sampse from Danish Hospital Institute, Knut Bernstein and Tove Lehrman from Danish Centre for Health Telematics. 1995

[8]   Impact of a large-scale health care network – the CoCo project. Knut Bernstein and Morten Bruun-Rasmussen from Danish Centre for Health Telematics, Giorgio Orsi and Luciana Ricciardiello from TSD Projects. 1998

[9]   Clinical Links Implementation Pack. NHS (England). 1997

[10] Dawes R M, Corrigan B, Linear models in decision making, Psychological Bulletin, 81: 95-106, 1974.

Heckerling P S, Elstein E S, Terzian C G, Kushner M S, The effect of incomplete knowledge on the diagnoses of a computer consultant system, Medical Informatics, 16: 363-370, 1991.

[11] The world's largest fair for medical equipment (primary, secondary, rehabilitation, laboratory) , drugs, hospital and practice infrastructure, publishers. http://www.tradefair.de/MEDICA98/D/index.htm

[12] CHIN Project 1996-1999, Co-operative Health Information Networks for the Community, HCT1007

[13] CHIN Project, Deliverable 22. March 1999

[14] TEN-ISDN Programme. European Commission. 1996

[15] Thomae Wirtschaftsforum, Ärzte-Betriebswirschaft 9/1997, S. 13 ff.

[16] Informations und Kommunikationsdienstegesctz v. 22.7. 1997, BGBl. I S. 1870

[17] Bundesarbeitsblatt 3/97, Verlag W. Kohlhammer, PraxiComputer Nr. 4, Sept. 1997, Datenschutz und Datensicherheit, Jahrgang 21, Heft 10, Oktober 1997

[18] Medonline, ISSN 0949-9059, MD-Verlags-GmbH Munich

[19] PRAXIS-Computer, a supplement to the "Deutsche Ärzteblatt" accessible also on-line at http://www.aezteblatt.de/

[20] Computerisation in GP Practices 1993 Survey. Department of Health NHS Management Executive, 1993.

[21] For Your Information: A Study of Information Management and Systems in the Acute Hospital. Audit Commission National Report, HMSO, London. 1995.

Appendix D

Description of six EU IVFP projects building RHCNs

A.1. Introduction

This appendix describes six EU IVth Framework Programme projects which are building RHCNs:

- CHIN;
- CoCo;
- Ithaca;
- Prestige;
- REMEDES;
- Star.

An introduction to the IVth Framework Programme is given, followed by an overview of the common themes for the projects described.

The following is described for each project:

- **Purpose of the project**

- **Regions participating in the project in general:** A short description of the regions participating in the project.

- **Regional partners in the RHCN build by the project:** A description of each "type" of Health Care Provider (partner) in the project - and the function and tasks the partners have in the regional health care system.

- **RHCN services provided by the project:** A description of each service in the RHCN: Information types covered, between which regional partners/users, motivation/benefits of partners, communication tasks, IT-service providers, usage scenario diagrams etc.

- **RHCN technical systems used in the project:** A description of the technical requirements and the technical way the RHCN is functioning: hardware and software, applications, standards, products, operational concepts, security issues, degree of integration with other systems etc.

- **RHCN products resulting from the project:** A description of long term business opportunities of the RHCN project-products, product candidates, problems, assessments by pilot users, cost-benefits etc.

- **Lessons learnt from project:** An assessment of the things learnt from the project, both good things and bad things; an assessment of the potential business case.

A.2. EU IVth Framework projects - introduction

In 1994, the Bangeman report "Europe and the global information society" recommended the creation of healthcare networks to promote less costly and more effective health care for Europe's citizens. The report states that a direct communication 'network of networks' is required, based on common standards, linking general practitioners, hospitals and social centres on a European scale. The role of the European Union, along with the member state health care systems, the insurance companies, the medical associations and the private sector is to promote standards and portable applications. It was envisaged that the citizen would benefit from improved diagnosis through on-line access to European specialists, on-line reservation of analysis and hospital services by practitioners etc. and that taxpayers and public administrations would benefit from tighter cost control and savings in healthcare spending and quicker reimbursement. The issue of safeguarding privacy and confidentiality of medical records was highlighted.

The Telematics Application Programme is one of the 19 specific programmes that are supported by the European Union's RTD IVth Framework Programme (1994 - 1998). It is a user driven research programme focusing on applications of information and/or communications technologies to society and is one of the building blocks for Europe's Information Society. The work of this programme impacts on a range of European policy areas such as health, education, transport and environment. The Telematics Applications Programme for the Health Care Sector is developing applications that help Europe's healthcare services meet people's expectations, through the efficient exchange of information between healthcare professionals, the transfer of medical records between remote sites and remote consultation. All of this will save time, money and lives, and improve clinical effectiveness, continuity and quality of care.

The IVth Framework Programme is currently supporting more than 100 projects concerning healthcare telematic applications, ranging from telematics assisted co-operative work for healthcare professionals and information for citizens, to tele-diagnosis, tele-consultation and emergency medicine. These projects are grouped into seven project groups in order to achieve the best possible synergy.

The Regional Health Care Network projects are in Group Four, which also contains the projects concerned with continuity of care and integration platforms. These projects have been grouped together to address the situation as it is today, and to move towards the achievement of a future vision which can be summarised as follows:

- Mobility: any healthcare professional can access any data about a specific patient in any place, subject to appropriate access rights, by facilities which enable them to connect to the network at any time.

- Integration: all systems are integrated in such a way that the end-user does not need to be concerned with different databases or formats and can easily access the information needed to provide care for the patient.

- Usability: The user interfaces to access patient data will be comprehensive and easy to use, requiring minimal training.

The current situation is that there are diverse solutions addressing isolated needs and tasks, often more directed to meeting the needs of administrators than healthcare professionals, and with limited integration. The role of integration platforms is to support the integration of discrete applications into an overall system dealing with information storage and exchange. However, integration platforms can be viewed as an intermediate solution, which will be replaced by emerging regional health care networks in the future.

To achieve continuity of care, data exchange is performed in two ways:

- exchange of standard messages e.g. EDIFACT, which does not imply a shared electronic patient record;
- the sharing of one unique or distributed electronic patient record from which the relevant information can be retrieved.

These two approaches are likely to coexist, at least for the foreseeable future, and the choice of solution is determined to some extent by organisational configurations. Ultimately, it is expected that this will be replaced by a shared/distributed electronic patient record on an inter/intranet based network, where patient confidentiality is controlled by adequate authorisation mechanisms which ensure that access to data for different actors is based on 'need to know' and patient consent.

The projects in Group Four and within the WISE project are addressing a range of technological and non-technological issues to move towards the vision outlined. This includes:

- the connection of different systems into one health care network;
- the development of intranet type solutions;
- the development of standards for data transmission;
- user acceptance;
- organisational change;
- regional policy;
- legal and security problems;
- the market.

A.3. EU projects on RHCNs

This section describes the common themes for RHCN based services, derived from the six IVth Framework Programme projects described in more details below. The section looks at the services provided by the projects, highlighting services common to more than one project.

The services provided by the IVth Framework Programme projects can be categorised as follows:

- clinical messages;
- sharing/integration of patient records;
- dissemination of health information, whether clinical information/protocols or health related information for the public.

In the context of RHCNs, there is another important category, administrative messages, which has not been addressed by these projects. These have been omitted largely because they are very specific to the healthcare system operated by each country, and there are therefore few opportunities for synergy between solutions for different countries. In addition, this area has often been the first addressed by national programmes.

In addition to these health specific services, RHCNs are routinely used for e-mail between the health professionals participating

A.3.1 *Clinical messages*

Clinical messages are used to exchange patient based clinical information, on what can be described as the "push" principle. That is, a clinician decides, on the basis of clinical need, that certain information about a patient needs to be sent to another person; different categories of information have different messages.

The clinical messages offered by these projects include the following:
- prescriptions;
- laboratory test request (or order);
- laboratory results reporting;
- diagnostic service (e.g. radiology, CAT, MRI, ultrasound, etc.) request (or order);
- diagnostic service (e.g. radiology, CAT, MRI, ultrasound, etc.) results reporting;
- referrals;
- hospitalisation request;
- hospital discharge summary;
- clinical balance during therapy (shared care).

All of these messages are characterised as follows:
- they contain patient identification;
- they contain clinical information, either (or both) coded and textual; coded information makes it easier for automated processing by the recipient;
- messages can be passed through a store-and-forward (e.g. e-mail like) network.

On-line Booking: Frequently associated with these clinical messages is an on-line appointment/outpatient booking activity. This is particularly true of referrals and diagnostic service requests. These involve many of the same healthcare actors, and very often similar data transfer requirements.

The various clinical messaging services implemented by the projects are shown in Figure D.1 below. This shows not only the store-and-forward services, but also the on-line booking service which is an important associated service.

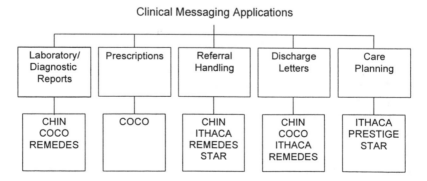

Figure D.1: Clinical messaging services

A.3.2 Sharing of patient records

In this category of services, patient information is exchanged through the "pull" principle. That is, clinicians are given access to patient information held on other systems.

These projects share data from patient records between different healthcare professionals involved in treating the patient, often from different organisations and locations. Rather than the approach of exchanging messages with clinical data described in above, here the approach is for healthcare professionals to be able to look at records held elsewhere (subject to security and privacy requirements).

This approach generally requires an on-line connection over a real-time network

The projects which have implemented services to share patient records are shown in Figure D.2 below. In the figure, Access to EHCR means read-only access to (a sub-set of) patient information, while Shared EHCR means a common patient record, often for a particular purpose, although the concept differs between projects, as does the method of achieving this. This also shows the on-line (appointment) booking service, as this requires an on-line network in a similar way to sharing of patient records.

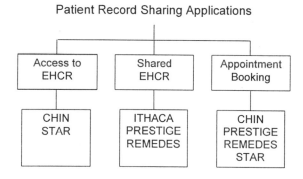

Figure D.2: Sharing of patient records

A.3.3 Health information

Dissemination of clinical information/protocols

These services disseminate information to clinical professionals. The information can be:
- clinical; for example, care protocols;
- in support of clinical processes; for example, costs, quality, waiting times, resource directories, statistical;
- global (national) in nature, or limited to a particular health organisation, or region.

These are typically on-line services, using for example internet web technology for managing the information dissemination.

While the information provided by these services does not come within the remit of the Data Protection Directive, it nevertheless may be sensitive to public scrutiny, and/or corruption. For example, it is essential that care protocols are only added and amended by authorised users. Therefore the network used need not, or even should not, be available to the general public. Private virtual networks, or encryption techniques, can be used to protect information from public scrutiny or amendment even if public networks are used.

Dissemination of health related information to the public

These services disseminate information to the general public, or subsets of it. The information can be:
- yellow pages of GPs, dentists, clinics etc.;
- public health information, and health education material.

The projects which have implemented services to disseminate health related information are shown in Figure D.3 below.

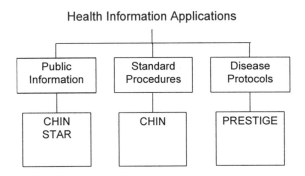

Figure D.3: Health information services

A.4. Co-operative Health Information Networks for the Community, CHIN

A.4.1 Purpose of the project

The CHIN initiative addresses the issue of establishing regional health information networks and focuses on information processes on the level of primary care. CHIN solutions are integrated in real working conditions of professionals and living conditions of citizens.

A.4.2 Regions participating in the project in general

CHIN is a collaborative enterprise of hospitals, physicians in private practices, healthcare administrations, universities and Information and Communications Technologies (ICT) industries involving seven nations (trial sites plus France). CHIN started project based operations in Athens/Lavrion/Kea (Greece), Berlin (Germany), Catalunya/Barcelona (Spain), North Karelia (Finland), Northern Sweden and Scotland. Figure D.4 illustrates the regional coverage of CHIN activities.

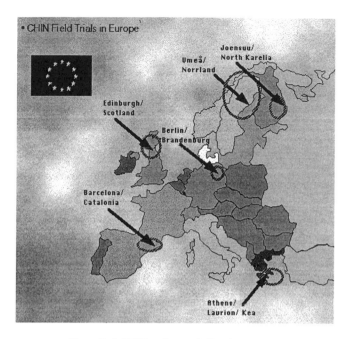

Figure D.4: CHIN regions and pilot sites

A.4.3 RHCN services provided by the project

CHIN covers a variety of Health Care Telematic Services (HCTS) which are based on a common IP-based technological concept and cost effective, standardised and flexible solutions. The HCTS implemented can be generally classified as services for healthcare professionals and on-line services for citizens/patients. The main objective was to show practically that HCTS assist doctors in improving their working processes with regard to interdisciplinary and inter-institutional co-operation, cost efficiency and total quality management and to enable citizens to easily retrieve information required to maintain their health and to utilise the healthcare services effectively. The variety of HCTS operated in different national European healthcare systems provide quantitative information on and indications as to how and where implementation of HCTS pays off.

Examples of CHIN healthcare services for professionals (CHIN-pro services) are remote access to multimedia patient records, quality control for screening results, referrals and resource planning, tele-pathology, tele-radiology, geographical health information systems, applications for diabetes care and mobile access to patient records for healthcare workers in remote areas of CHIN pilot sites. In addition, requirements for professional, non-patient related on-line information are covered, e.g. for education or administration. As one example, Figure D.5 shows screen shots of a Web-based multimedia patient record. The information displayed represents a dynamically updated HTML-based virtual meta-patient record, whereby the information items are being retrieved via a specific meta-patient record database with interfaces to the Web and information subsystems (e.g. imaging equipment, archives etc.). These systems allow the logical integration of physically distributed patient (and other) data which can be accessed by authorised personnel via intranet, Figure D.6.

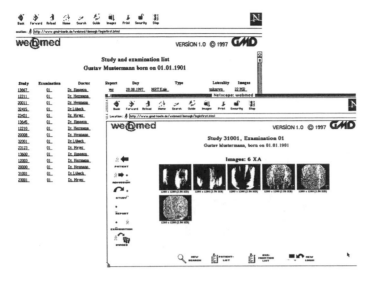

Figure D.5: Patient data integration via Web and HTML

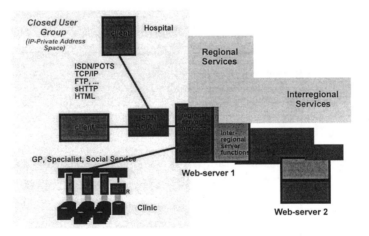

Figure D.6: ISDN based intranet, interfaces to the internet

The CHIN services for public access include web-based regional healthcare resource directories - a presentation platform for regional healthcare service providers - on-line information for health education (both for professionals and citizens) and references to web-sites found useful by CHIN members systematically ordered. Figure D.7 and Figure D.8 show elements of the CHIN public sites of Scotland.

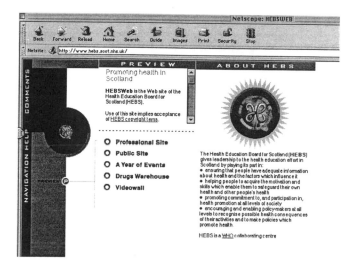

Figure D.7: CHIN-public services: Health Education Board Scotland (HEBS).

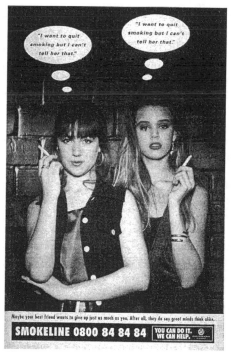

Figure D.8: HEBS: an education page for juvenile.

All public sites are designed according to one design concept, information necessary to navigate through the sites is available in several languages and if information changes frequently, there is a web-data-base interface to guarantee up to date information, Figure D.9.

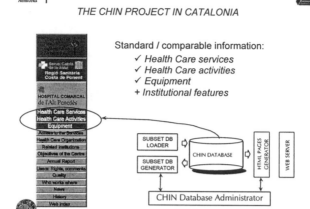

Figure D.9: Active CHIN web-sites with DB-Web-interfaces.

A.4.4 RHCN technical systems used in the project

Technically, CHIN favours standardised, simple, open and scaleable solutions for the medical applications (DICOM, HL7) as well as regarding computer and networking technologies (ISDN based intranets, HTTP). IP protocols and the Web are the general communication platform. Access via analogue telephone networks is also supported. Security mechanisms are implemented for CHIN pro-services depending on the specific requirements. Access to CHIN information resources is practically possible from any place having access to the internet. In the case of patient related or other confidential information, access is only possible for authorised personnel based on person roles and a security concept set up by the HCTS operators.

A CHIN extension is foreseen which will provide access to filtered CHIN and CHIN-like information via mobile end-systems such as PDAs or notebook computers using GSM and satellite networks (including next generation satellite systems such as MEO - Medium Earth Orbit Satellites - and LEO - Low Earth Orbit Satellites). Specific information services tailored to suit the information needs of mobile healthcare workers and citizens of developing countries are included. Access to CHIN or CHIN-like information will be possible via mobile end-systems and GSM or satellite

Further information and examples of public and professional services can be found under http://b5www.berkom.de/CHIN/

A.5. CoCo

A.5.1 Purpose of the CoCo project

The objective of CoCo is to improve the co-ordination and continuity of health care and social services. This is done by establishing pilots of RHCNs in 10 regions in 8 European countries. In parallel with the technological implementation, business process re-engineering (BPR) in the participating organisations is guided and supported. Project "ownership" by the users - the regions - is one key element in CoCo. This will ensure committed participation from the users and the continuous focus on real user needs.

Once this regional health care data network has been established, the communication will be of such size that operations and further developments are expected to continue under normal commercial conditions.

CoCo will result in European added value in three important areas:

1. The implementation guidelines, handbooks, BPR guidelines, evaluation models and computer tools used and validated in CoCo, can be immediately applied in other implementation projects.

2. The emerging CEN standards (and other standards) will be validated on a large scale, providing important feed-back to other European standardisation efforts.

3. The Regional Health Care Networks are expected to be exploited on a commercial basis after the project, and CoCo therefore strongly supports the European market for telematics services in health care.

CoCo paves the way for other implementation projects and supports dissemination of the technology throughout Europe. This implies a better service for patients, higher professional standards and a more efficient health care sector.

A.5.2 Regions participating in the project in general

The CoCo contractors are:
- County of Funen (DK)
- South and East Belfast Health & Social Services Trust (UK)
- North Western and North Eastern Health Boards (EI)
- Consorci Hospitalari de Catalunya (SP)
- Norwegian Centre for Medical Informatics (NO)
- Hellenic Committee for HOPE Programme (GR)
- Erasmus University (NL)
- TSD-Projects Srl (IT)
- Azienda USSL12 di Bergamo (IT)
- Ipswich General Hospital NHS Trust (UK)
- Prince Edward Island Health and Community Services (CAN)

The CoCo regions are technically, financially and organisationally self-contained. The regional authorities are fully responsible for developing their own health care data network in the region, focusing on their own needs and interests - but supported by the CoCo-Link activities

The knowledge transfer from the link activities is produced by the most experienced participants within different areas. In CoCo they are responsible for producing guides and supporting other regions in building regional healthcare networks.

Appendix D

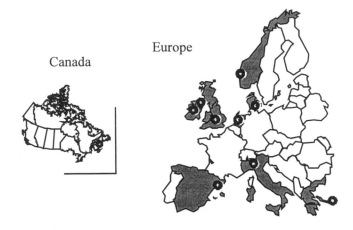

Figure D.10: Contractors in the CoCo project by country

The major partners on CoCo are mainly regional/national healthcare authorities, who want to implement their own regional healthcare networks. In Denmark, Norway, Ireland and Spain, the national authorities support the projects; that is, the test sites which are included in CoCo are selected as national test-sites. In Northern Ireland, England, The Netherlands, Italy and Greece, CoCo includes regional projects with support from regional or national authorities. Several regions are already highly experienced in EDI development and large scale validation.

CoCo is a large project. In total it is planned that 24 hospitals and more than 230 GP clinics participate.

A.5.3 Regional partners in the RHCN built by the project

Due to specialisation of the healthcare system, many different providers are involved in the service for a patient during the patient's episode of care. Thus, there is extensive communication between the different participants of the healthcare sector. The starting point for electronic communication was the most frequent and resource demanding messages. The GP offices receive laboratory results and discharge letters from the hospitals and general hospital information (e.g. waiting list figures) from the county administration. The GP sends prescriptions to the pharmacies and reimbursement claims to the county administration.

On average, each hour of consultation with the general practitioner (GP) results in more than one message to another part of the healthcare sector. This generates a large flow of routine messages, such as prescriptions, referrals, examination requests, discharge letters and laboratory results. In the Netherlands, 300 million messages are exchanged annually. When adding to this the reimbursement communications (which makes up about one-third of the medical data), the total number of messages exceeds the communication in, for example, the financial sector.

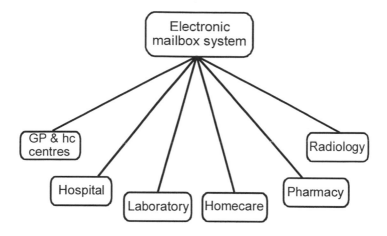

Figure D.11: Partners in the health care data network

Because of specialisation and division of labour, there is a need for extensive communication between the participants involved in the healthcare sector. Everyday routine messages include prescriptions, referrals, discharge letters and laboratory results. There is also a growing need for new information on home care, use of images, access to quality databases, exchange of health care records, etc.

The accurate, fast and safe communication of information has, therefore, become decisive to the cost, quality and patient service of the entire health service. The traditional manner of printing data from one computer system, sending it by mail, and finally typing the same information into another system, counteracts these goals.

The CoCo project addresses these challenges of the fragmented health care sector by offering widespread use of Telematics and simultaneously supports re-engineering of the work processes.

To integrate the IT systems in healthcare, CoCo establishes regional networks between the most important parts of the healthcare sector. CoCo uses existing technology and common European pre-CEN standards for the most frequent messages used in primary health care.

In short: CoCo is making standardised EDI (Electronic Data Interchange) in European healthcare, involving all health and social care professionals in their daily work.

A.5.4 RHCN services provided by the project

The messages sent by the healthcare network consist first and foremost of prescriptions, hospital discharge letters, referrals, laboratory reports and radiology reports.

Prescriptions: The electronic prescriptions replace not only the hand-written prescriptions but also those which the doctor telephones directly to the pharmacy. The electronic prescriptions is routed directly into the pharmacy's computer system for further processing. This method of handling prescriptions saves time and reduces the risk of errors.

Discharge letters: Hospital discharge letters are an important piece of information from the hospital to the GP in connection with the discharge of a patient. Traditionally, there has been a problem in that these discharge letters took to long in making their way to the GP. After the establishment of the healthcare network, the discharge letter on average arrives at the GP eight days earlier than before. This improvement in time is not just due to the electronic communication, but is also due to the modification in procedures that have come about due to implementation of the network.

Laboratory reports: Rapid and precise communication of the results of laboratory analyses are important for patient treatment. Within this area, a large number of laboratory reports can be transferred automatically from machine to machine every day by the healthcare network. Laboratory reports include reports from the pathology departments, the clinical biochemistry departments and the microbiological departments. The time savings compared with sending the analysis reports by mail is typically one day.

Radiology Reports: Results on radiological investigations are also transferred from radiology departments to the GPs by the healthcare network.

Referrals: Referrals from GPs to hospitals and specialist doctors become more precise when they are filled out electronically and sent by the healthcare network. Before being able to sent referral electronically, it is necessary to agree on the information to be sent. The referral can only be sent if all information is present.

Hospital Information: Current information on the occupancy of hospital departments, waiting times, treatment procedures etc., are important information for the GP when advising the patient. The information on the hospitals is collected, edited and sent electronically to GPs.

Other communication to primary care: Variants of the standards can be used for a series of other messages: Nursing reports to the home care nurse, request and results to physiotherapy, shared care protocols, booking, etc.

Multimedia messages : CoCo also develops systems for communication of messages with multimedia content, such as images, ECGs, graphics from laboratories, etc. The technology is parallel to that used for text based messages. This means that a GP for example can communicate all kind of messages from the same workstation - the converter/gateway takes care of wrapping and sending the messages the correct way.

A.5.5 RHCN technical systems used in the project

The basic idea of CoCo is to send structured electronic messages from one computer to another for healthcare communication. This means that data entered once can be re-used elsewhere in the sector. To make this EDI (Electronic Data Interchange) work, standards for the communication format are needed. CoCo has developed most of the messages on the basis of the EDIFACT message standard. To make it easier for the developers in the regions to build EDIFACT message communication facilities into their application, CoCo is delivering several tools and guidelines for use in the regions. When the standards and the applications are in place, messages can start to flow in the Regional Health Care Network. Most regions base their network on an electronic mailbox system.

Thus, CoCo is not inventing new technology. On the contrary, CoCo is building on existing applications, the infrastructure most appropriate in the specific situation (i.e. normal telephone lines, ISDN, ATM etc.), European standardisation work, and well known mailbox techniques. In CoCo this is customised for healthcare, implemented and validated in new regional networks - in a non-mature marketplace.

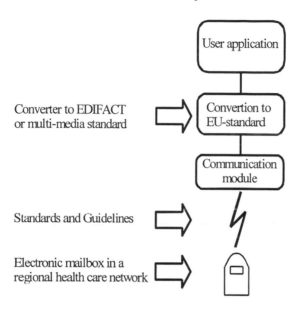

Figure D.12: The basic technology used in CoCo

One important part of the integration technology comprises a regional mailbox system. The mailbox may be a store-and-forward system from a VANS operator, an internet based system, etc. The mailbox system is the hub of the information system. It works in the same way as the routine e-mail system: from the mailbox, each participant (physician, laboratory, hospital) receives their personal mail, and from the same mailbox messages are sent to other parties. Encrypting the messages is also possible if required, and this will also be validated in some CoCo pilots.

Unlike many other integration methods, the mailbox system works 24 hours a day, even if the recipient's computer system is not active. The mailbox system is highly suited to standardisation using messages.

The participants have computer systems from different vendors, but the Regional Health Care Networks together with the developed standards makes electronic communication between the systems possible. The idea is to exchange structured information, which can be understood and re-used in the receiving system. European EDIFACT standards have been selected for the communication.

Many health and social care professionals have today access to computer systems, but often they do not have the right software to support the way of working. Maybe the software is not developed yet, or the organisation is too small to pay the expenses for the software, implementation and education.

In the past years, the use of internet has increased explosively. The internet is an easy and low cost way to send data, but the need for defining standards messages still exists, independently from the specific network and protocol implementations that will be selected and adopted.

In CoCo, a system based on EDI and internet has been implemented. The target group for the system is small users who have a low volume of messages and do not have software and communication capabilities. To run the system you only need a access to the Internet. If messages are send in EDIFACT format to a user of the new system, the EDIFACT message is automatically stored in a database and converted to HTML. This means that the user can view the information with a standard browser. The application also contains functionality, for instance to view different types of incoming messages and check for who has accessed the documents.

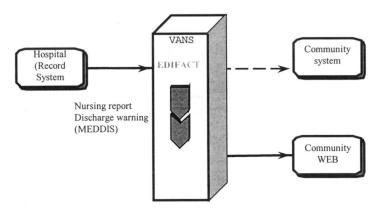

Figure D.13: EDI and internet

As an example, the system is used when the hospital nurse wants to alert the home care nurse that the patient will soon be discharged or if she wants to send a nursing report at the time of discharge. The electronic patient record system converts the information to EDIFACT format, and the message is sent to the electronic mailbox as usual. If a community system can handle EDIFACT, they fetch the mail as usual. Most community systems do not handle EDIFACT; in these cases, the information can be looked up at a password protected part of the community web.

A.5.6 RHCN products resulting from the project

CoCo delivers everything which is needed to build a regional health care network:
- standards for communication based on CEN TC251;
- tools for testing regional standards and integration with existing software;
- BPR guidelines and toolkit;
- validation methodology;
- training, standards and BPR.

To make it possible for the participating software providers to develop their applications, CoCo produces several EDIFACT standards for the selected messages.

For each message, a CoCo Standard is produced in a "European version"; these can be used by the regions to make their own regional Message Implementation Guides (MIG). These European CoCo standards will be produced following the pre-standardisation work done by CEN (WG3) and EBES(EEG9), but taking as a starting point the national MIGs already produced in UK, Norway and Denmark.

Two types of EDI tools are produced to help the regional software providers in implementing their EDI standards: a CoCo Converter and a CoCo simulator; both take their starting point in already existing software products in this area.

The converter is distributed to the region's software suppliers. The converter has the regional CoCo standards built in. The EDI Converter is a software product; it is similar to other EDI converters, but is configured to communicate the CoCo EDIFACT messages (MEDREF, MEDDIS, HOME CARE etc.).

Another aspect of the integration system is the establishment of communication functionality in the existing computer systems in the region, e.g. in the physician's electronic health care record and hospital's Patient Administration System. This requires two standard elements: an EDI converter and a communication module.

An EDI converter is delivered to the suppliers from CoCo. Each application supplier must then develop an interface between his own database and the EDI converter. This interface can be developed by the supplier on the basis of the CoCo guidelines and local expertise.

CoCo also delivers a testing tool called an EDIFACT Simulator. This tool is a help for developer when implementing EDIFACT communication functionality in their systems.

The benefits expected from the coherent and synergetic implementation of all the mentioned projects can be listed as follows:
- improvement in the quality of services provided;
- improved accessibility to healthcare services for citizens;
- simplification of procedures, both for citizens and professionals;
- integration of primary and secondary care/social assistance;
- more accurate results and faster results availability.

A.5.7 Lessons learnt from project

From the management and technical point of view, advice can be given on the following five points:

1. Make a good survey for the current running systems in region. If there are missing systems or functionality, it will prevent the dissemination of the communication. Do not investigate only the number of users with computers, but include the software and examine how the system supports the daily work.

2. Do not only take the benefits from changing to electronic communication, but use the opportunity to change the organisation and make analyses of the current workflow in the organisation.

3. Make sure their is full commitment from the local health authorities, and involve all healthcare organisations and associations in the project.

4. The semantics part of the data to be transferred is the difficult part. Do not underestimate this work. Establish groups with members from different users, vendors and healthcare authorities, and get small pilots running before dissemination. The result of the semantics work can be used later on in the implementation phase, independent of the type of standards.

5. Establish test nodes, for instance with some of the developers of the receiving software, where the messages can be tested in a formalised way.

In addition, the Danish Hospital Institute has performed an evaluation of the regional health care network in the County of Funen (FynCom). The evaluation was mainly based on a survey. Questionnaires were sent to 22 general practice offices in Funen County of which 18 responded, to 23 clinical departments of which 20 responded, and to 9 laboratories of which 6 responded. Two pharmacists and several key persons who took part in the initiation and implementation of the system were also interviewed. In addition, literature, statistical material, minutes of meetings etc. were studied. The general approach of the evaluation was that of technology assessment.

Many different aspects was evaluated. Technical aspects, user-friendliness of the systems, security, organisational aspects in the hospitals etc. will not be discussed here. This paper will focus on the time savings and economic aspects at the GPs.

Organisational changes were a prerequisite as well as a consequence of the introduction of FynCom. In 10 of the 18 practices, division of labour between the physician and his secretary had changed, mostly with slightly more communication work to the physician and much less to the secretary. Except for prescriptions, mainly physicians operate FynCom.

The time saving for an average general practice (2.3 physicians) with a daily administration of 26 prescriptions, 3 laboratory replies, 2 discharge letters and general hospital information was more than 50 minutes per day, or 22 minutes per physician.

Patient service was improved due to the faster response rate. On average the GP could present the discharge letter to the patient 8.2 days earlier than with traditional means of communication, and the laboratory reply was available one day earlier. For the patient this means more timely information, less uncertainty and possibility of prompt initiation of after-treatment, which can reduce morbidity and absence from work.

A.6. Ithaca

A.6.1 Purpose of the project

The aim of ITHACA is to improve the quality of care provided to people living in the community through the integration and validation of telematic services capable of supporting the efficient sharing of relevant information between health and social care professionals.

A.6.2 Regions participating in the project in general

A.6.2.1 South & East Belfast, Northern Ireland

The South & East Belfast region is an area within the city of Belfast with a population of just over 200.000 people and 95.000 households.

South & East Belfast Health & Social Services Trust (SEBT) is the co-ordinating partner for ITHACA and provides community health and social care for the South & East Belfast region. The Trust works in close collaboration and liaison with General Practitioners who are independent contractors. The 46 GP practices in the South & East Belfast region act as gatekeepers in the health care system, i.e. they are responsible for referring eligible patients to secondary care.

Secondary care is provided by five general hospitals and seven specialised hospitals (two maternity, one children's, one fever/cancer, one psychiatric and one elderly) – these also serve other regions within Northern Ireland.

The regional partners are:
- South & East Belfast Health & Social Services Trust;
- Systems Team Group - developer of the ITHACA demonstrator for Belfast, to be validated at most other sites;
- Ordnance Survey, Northern Ireland – developer of a GIS demonstrator for ITHACA.

A.6.2.2 Andalucia, Spain

The Andalucia region in Spain has a population of some 7.000.000 people. Servicio Andaluz de Salud (SAS) is the regional health authority for Andalucia and a contractor in ITHACA.

The regional partners are:
- Servicio Andaluz de Salud;
- Empresa Publica Hospital Costa del Sol - secondary care hospital involved in demonstration;
- Ingenieria e Integracion Avanzadas - developer of a maternal health demonstrator;
- Prodimed - developer of a child health demonstrator;
- Universidad Politecnica de Madrid - developer of a home telecare demonstrator.

A.6.2.3 Municipality of Turku, Finland

The Municipality of Turku has a population of approximately 160.000 people. The ITHACA contractor in the region is the Health Office, City of Turku, which is responsible for the provision of services in health and social care.

The regional partners are:
- Health Office, City of Turku;
- Tiedonhallinta Oy – developer of a demonstrator for Turku;

- VTT Technology – to contribute to functional specifications.

A.6.2.4 Porto, Portugal

The Porto sub-region is part of the Regional Health Authority for Northern Portugal and provides healthcare to a population of 500.000. The Regional Health Authority is a contractor in ITHACA.

The regional partners are:
- Administracao Regional de Saude do Norte;
- Instituto de Engenharia de Sistemas e Computadores – developer of demonstrator for Porto;
- Maternidade de Julio Dinis – maternity hospital involved in pilot;
- Magalhaes Lemos Hospital – mental hospital involved in pilot.

A.6.2.5 Oise Region, France

FACSSO is a federation of organisations co-ordinating community health and social care for the elderly and disabled. The area covered by FACSSO has a population of 350.000 people.

The regional partners are:
- Federation des Associations de Coordination Sanitaire et Sociale de L'Oise.

A.6.2.6 Bergamo (Lombardy Region), Italy

The district of Bergamo has a population of 380.000. Health care services are provided by USSL12. There are four hospitals, 10 health centres and almost 450 GPs in the district

The regional partners are:
- Azienda USSL 12;
- TSD Projects – provides technical support to USSL12.

A.6.2.7 Municipality of Amaroussion, Athens, Greece

The Municipality of Amaroussion has a population of 100.000 and provides municipal services including health and social services.

The regional partners are:
- National Technical University of Athens – has responsibility for functional specifications and technical support to the other partners in Greece;
- Hellenic Red Cross – involved in pilot with Municipality of Amaroussion.

A.6.2.8 Gothenburg, Sweden

The area involved in ITHACA is the Community Unit of Orgryte, which has a population of 30,.000 of which over 30% are over 65 years of age. The unit is responsible for child care, leisure, culture, care of the handicapped, family care and senior citizen care programmes.

The regional partners are:

- City Council of Gothenburg, Orgryte Community Unit;
- SDN–Data – provides technical support to Orgryte Community Unit.

A.6.2.9 Dublin, Ireland & Cavan/Monaghan, Ireland

The area of the Eastern Health Board has a population of 1,23 million. The unit involved in ITHACA is the Clondalkin Mental Health Service which is responsible for providing a comprehensive community based mental health service to a population of around 60.000.

The area of Cavan, Monaghan, Louth and Meath are covered by the North Western Health Board. In ITHACA, the West Cavan District and Cavan/Monaghan Services for the Elderly are involved. This covers an area of around 26.000 inhabitants with 15% over 65 years of age.

The regional partners are:
- Irish Medical Systems – provides technical support to Irish sites;
- Eastern Health Board;
- North Eastern Health Board.

A.6.2.10 Saskatchewan, Canada

The province of Saskatchewan is in the process of reforming its health system to be client centred with a focus on wellness and community based services. Saskatchewan Health are partners in the project because of the similarities between the approach in ITHACA to the development of their client-centred integrated care management information system, allowing opportunities for valuable collaboration in a number of areas.

A.6.3 Regional partners in the RHCN build by the project

Regional Health Authorities: Have the responsibility for the provision and co-ordination of health services including financial management of services.

Community Health and Social Care Providers: Provide a range of health services including district nursing; health visiting; podiatry; physiotherapy; occupational therapy; speech and language therapy; psychology; psychotherapy and mental health services. A range of home care services is provided as well as health care within sheltered dwellings and day care centres.

General Hospitals: Provide a range of secondary care for all client groups.

Maternity Hospitals: Provide maternal care to women and a referral service from perinatal hospitals.

Psychiatric Hospitals: Provide acute mental health services – in-patient and day hospital psychiatric care.

A.6.4 RHCN services provided by the project

1. WEBinfo: General information concerning treatment, costs, quality, waiting times etc.
2. Statistics: Statistical reporting to other partners.

3. Guides: Clinical guideline for co-operative care on selected diseases.
4. Research: Retrieving research and statistics from databases from other partners.
5. E-mail: Transfer of an unstructured textual message of different kind from one partner.
6. Prescription: Transfer of prescription to pharmacy.
7. Referral: Transfer of referral to another partner in RHC.
8. Discharge: Transfer of discharge-information from hospital.
9. Lab-result: Transfer of laboratory result from a laboratory.
10. X-ray result: Transfer of X-ray or X-ray description from radiology clinic.
11. Protocol: Transferring information used in "shared care" between the partners.
12. Records: Patient record - send to another partner.
13. EKG: EKG-results send to another partner.
14. Ordering: Transfer an order to another partner.
15. Telecare: Transfer an alert message from a device in client's home to a partner
16. Telemonitoring Transfer an alert message from a device on client's body to a partner
17. Assign_From: Assign a resource/service from a partner
18. Assign_To Assign a Resource/service to a partner
19. Transfer Care Plan to another partner
20. Transfer Intervention History to another partner
21. Transfer Client history to another partner (medical/social/psychiatric etc history)
22. Transfer Investigation Result (ASCII) to another partner (eg Lab_Result)
23. Transfer Investigation Result (Multimedia) to another partner (eg ECG, EEG, x-ray, ultrasound scan)
24. Booking: Booking of appointment for treatment or investigations.
25. Telnet: Remote terminal access to patient record systems.

A.6.4.1 Motivation/benefits of partners

- The anticipated benefits for software companies of the generic system are maintainability and marketability.

- The system should support person centred care.

- The system should support multidisciplinary sharing of information for professionals working at different locations.

- The benefits of the generic core across client groups is anticipated to be better information on cases which fall into more than one client group e.g. elderly and mental health.

- The system should provide better statistical information for managing the service.

- The accuracy of the information held on the system should be better than for current information systems, assisted by easier data input and less duplication.

- Professionals should have access to more complete information enabling them to provide better quality care.

- The system should prompt reengineering of services.

- It should lead to better decision-making, better planning of care, better information in an emergency, and better identification of risk.

- The system should improve access to services for patients and greater choice.

A.6.5 RHCN technical systems used in the project

A.6.5.1 Networking/platforms

With regard to the types of network supporting ITHACA services at the various sites, a variety of networking protocols have been adopted according to the local site infrastructures. These are :

- TCP/IP (Transport Control Protocol / Internet Protocol)
- SNMP Network Management (Simple Network Management Protocol). Recommended
- ODI Novell(Open data-link interface)
- NDIS (Network Device Interface Specification)
- ISDN Bridge (Integrated Services Digital Network)
  For Dial-Up Remote Access :
- PPP (Point to Point Protocol)

Server Operating Systems:

- UNIX SVR4
- Windows NT (XPG3)
- Novell

Client Operating Systems used:

- OS/2
- Windows 95
- Windows NT

Application communication mechanisms used:

- DDE (Dynamic Data Exchange)
- OLE (Object Linking and Embedding)
- NET DDE
- CORBA (Common Object Request Broker Architecture)

A.6.5.2 Development tools

Development tools for Windows 95:

- Visual Basic
- Visual C++
- Delphi
- PowerBuilder

Development standards and approach:

- Generic application design through the application of an Object-oriented analysis and design methodology (Rumbaugh & Jacobsen). Tools: Rational Rose and Select Enterprise.

- Consistent user interface across the various development sites : This aim was partially achieved, compromised to some extent by the need to integrate ITHACA services with those provided by other systems at client sites.

- Database independence of resulting prototypes - can be implemented on any ODBC-compliant database.

A.6.5.3 Applications

Operational clinical management systems with a generic design enabling adaptation of the services to the operational needs of any community health provider. This aim was tested by implementing the ITHACA prototypes for each of the following client groups:
- maternal and child care;
- elderly care information management system;
- mental health.

A.6.5.4 Products

D3.1 – Methodology for User Requirements
D3.2 – User Requirements
D4.1 – High Level Functional Specification
D4.2 – Detailed Functional Specification
D4.3 – Definition of Demonstrators
D5.1 – Survey of Existing Technologies
D5.4 – Application Software for Assessment, Care Planning and to Support Delivery of Care
D5.5 – Optimisation tools Application Software
D5.6 – Client Tools Application Software
D6.1 – Installation Plans
D6.2 – Training Plans (Demonstrator Sites)
D7.1/2 – Verification Methodology, Plans and Scenarios
D7.3 – Verification Report
D8.1 – Preliminary Evaluation Report
D8.2 – Final Evaluation Report

A.6.5.5 Security issues

ITHACA has addressed security issues from the perspective of the requirements of health care providers; which kinds of information can be shared, at what level, and definition of the team structures into which security constraints are to be applied. This was a particular requirement for those ITHACA sites working with mental health teams – Belfast, Turku and Porto.

The technical implementation options to meet those requirements were outside the scope of ITHACA, each ITHACA pilot site implemented its security protocol according to the local technical infrastructure.

A.6.5.6 Integration with other systems

All of the services provided by ITHACA prototypes have been developed on the basis of a common generic design using object-oriented methods. The project found a high degree of convergence in the definition of ideal healthcare processes across countries and across client groups, so the prototypes were developed to facilitate those processes. For this reason, a high degree of commonality between prototypes was envisaged, and early indications are that this has been partially achieved in ITHACA, with some compromises. The challenge faced by the ITHACA development sites was the need to integrate their prototypes into a pre-existing local infrastructure, whilst remaining true to the generic design and generic user interface components.

Integration of prototypes with other systems - examples:
- Belfast - with community resource management system
- Porto - with SINUS and SONHO hospital information systems

A.6.6 RHCN products resulting from the project

ITHACA has already provided significant business benefit to the participating healthcare organisations and companies from the following perspectives.

For healthcare organisations, there is now a reference model that can be used for the evaluation of any local healthcare procedure, facilitating the identification of "best practice" and supporting the endeavour of re-engineering healthcare processes where appropriate.

For companies, an analysis model which has been tested across Europe and across diverse client group requirements; this has provided invaluable research information for those companies considering trans-national marketing and implementation of those systems.

A.6.7 Lessons learnt from the project

It is too early to attempt to describe the lessons learnt, since the validation phase has not yet been completed. An important achievement has been the development of the model for health and social care processes, applicable across sites and client groups. Early feedback indicates that the demonstrators developed from this model will make a significant contribution to the benefits anticipated by health care providers.

A.7. PRESTIGE

A.7.1 Purpose of the project

The main purpose of *PRESTIGE* is to deliver an installed and sustainable healthcare telematics infrastructure that supports the generation, dissemination and application of research-based and consensus-based guidelines defining best practice in clinical care.

The overall project structure is shown in the figure below. This structure forms the basic architecture for the interaction between clinical scenarios and technology. The activities in cardiology, cancer, diabetes and neurology are implementing support for computerised guidelines in both primary care and hospital settings, in each case addressing problems of co-operative and shared care between these sectors.

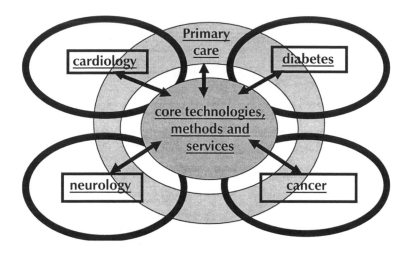

Figure D.14 - *PRESTIGE* structure

Substantial user involvement has been assured through national and specialist user groups and renowned healthcare centres. *PRESTIGE* is making available a common pool of interoperable technologies to these user groups and clinical sites in the following areas:

- architectures for multimedia patient records
- act management
- terminology and multilingual services
- generic models for representing guidelines and protocols.

A.7.2 Regions participating in the project in general

Key health regions involved in the project include:

A.7.2.1 Health Region of Lisboa and Tejo Valley, Portugal

The Health Region of Lisboa and Tejo Valley (population 3.564.768) comprises the sub-regions of Lisboa, Setúbal and Santarém. The sub-region of Lisboa (population 2.351.901) is divided in six Health Units which aggregate the services provided by primary and secondary / tertiary care. Prestige activities are centred in the Health Unit C of Lisboa (population 446.700).

In Portugal, provision of healthcare services is mainly dependent on a National Health System complemented by a set of sub-systems, private services, and a small number of health insurance systems. It follows a summary of the role played by the key organisations involved in the healthcare process in a health region:

- Health Region Administrations (ARS) have the responsibility in co-ordinating all healthcare organisations within the territory they are responsible, including the definition of healthcare policies. The Health Region Administration of Lisboa and Tejo Valley is a partner in *PRESTIGE*.

- Primary care Health Centres (PCHC) are the key element of the healthcare system, and are under the direct administration of ARS bodies. Centro Saude

Ajuda (CSA) is the primary care health centre (population 31.000) directly involved in *PRESTIGE* activities.

- Hospitals, provide specialised services to citizens; hospitals are usually classified according to their degree of specialisation and the population they serve, i.e. district, central, university, etc.. Hospitals have their own budget, in part derived from direct billing to healthcare sub-systems, in part funded through the PNP. Hospital Egas Moniz (HEM), a partner to *PRESTIGE*, is the main central hospital of the Health Unit C, hence serving all the population of the Health Unit C.

A.7.2.2 Modena Health Unit, Italy

The Modena Local Health Unit Enterprise (Azienda Unità Sanitaria Locale di Modena), a partner to *PRESTIGE*, represents one of the 13 local health authorities of Emilia-Romagna Region (3,9 million inhabitants) of North-Italy. It covers an area representing the whole Province (613.000 inhabitants). It was created in 1994 as consequence of the combination of the 6 previous local health units by the application of the new law concerning national health re-organisation. With a density of 228 inhabitants/km2 (v. 178 of E-R region, or v. 188 of Italy) it is the second most populated health local unit in Italy.

A.7.2.3 County of Funen, Denmark

The County of Funen is located almost at the centre of Denmark. The county consist of a larger island called Funen and a number of smaller islands surrounding it. Funen is connected to Jutland and Sealand by bridges (The last one opened in June 1998, the worlds second largest suspension bridge).

The main city is Odense, approximately 185.000 inhabitants. In the coastal area there are 8 - 10 cities ranging from small to middle-sized, approximately from 5.000 to 40.000 inhabitants. There are approximately 475.000 inhabitants in the County of Funen. The number of inhabitants in the urban areas of Funen comes to approximately 350.000. This means that the rural area will account for approximately 125.000 inhabitants.

Figure D.15 below shows a map of the County of Funen with the major cities. Odense is the main city. Odense University Hospital (OUH) is located here; this is a tertiary care facility, with 1300 beds. In organisational terms, there is also one secondary care facility called Sygehus Fyn. However this secondary care facility consists of 9 smaller hospitals ranging from 50 to 250 beds; until recently, these were individual organisations. One of these secondary care hospitals is located in each of the other cities shown. All are connected via the County network, Frame-relay

The number of General Practitioners is approximately 315 and the number of practising specialists comes to around 60, making a total of 375 doctors.

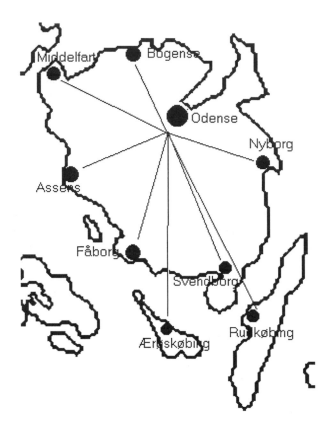

Figure D.15: The County of Funen

Partners in the Danish *PRESTIGE* project are Odense University Hospital, which will act as a tertiary care facility, while Sygehus Fyn Middelfart, Assens, Svendborg, Ærøskøbing, Rudkøbing, Fåborg, Nyborg and Bogense will act as secondary care facilities. There will also be a number of general practices involved, that refer patients to these hospitals. Ramboll (MediCare) will act as a general practice systems supplier.

A.7.2.4 Other regions involved in the project

PRESTIGE concepts are being demonstrated through application pilots in specific clinical specialities by means of the participation in the project of a variety of health care organisations, in several European countries. A description of the type and functions of these project partners is provided in the next section below in terms of the different project actions implemented.

The following health care regions are in this context also indirectly involved in the project:
- North Thames Region, UK.
- Sowerby Unit, Northern Region, UK.
- Trent region, UK

A.7.3 Regional partners in the RHCN build by the project

PRESTIGE is structured into several actions (e.g. application sub-projects) addressing major healthcare specialities including cardiothoracic disease, neurological disease, diabetes and general practice. It follows a brief description of the healthcare providers in the project in terms of the guidelines being implemented in the different healthcare specialities represented in the project.

A.7.3.1 Cardiology

The Cardiology Sub-Project in *PRESTIGE* is split into three clinical scenarios
- Shared Care for Heart Disease, in UK;
- Hospital Care for Heart Disease, in Germany;
- Shared Care Anticoagulant Therapy, in Denmark.

A.7.3.1.1 Shared Care for Heart Disease

The objective in this scenario is to implement protocol directed shared care for the management of coronary artery disease across General Practices, District General Hospitals and the Royal Brompton Hospital as a Specialist Centre. The partners (healthcare providers) involved are Royal Brompton Hospital, Bromley Hospital, Chelsea and Westminster Hospital within the North Thames Region, UK.

A.7.3.1.2 Hospital Care for Heart Disease

The objective of this scenario is to implement protocol directed shared care for the management of coronary artery disease in the 2nd Medical Clinic of the Mainz Heart Centre at Johannes Gutenbert-University in Mainz. In particular Mainz concentrates on the workflow surrounding patient management in the catheter laboratory and on this model a multimedia document based application is being built to support protocol directed care.

A.7.3.1.3 Shared Care Anticoagulant Therapy

This scenario is concerned with management of patients on Anticoagulant Therapy across general practices, district general hospitals/secondary care facilities, clinical chemistry laboratories and tertiary care facilities. The Danish cardiology scenario of ACT in the context of *PRESTIGE* relates closely to a Danish project called THROMBO-Base. The objective of THROMBO-Base is to improve quality of maintenance ACT using several different forms of information technology, one of which is guideline interacting with the electronic patient record used. Key partners (healthcare providers) involved are the Danish Institute for Health Services DK (DSI), and the Department of Clinical Chemistry County of Funen, DK (FUNEN).

During the project, a computer front-end, an EDIFACT message and a clinical database will be developed. The computer front-end is based on the Danish National Guideline for Anticoagulant Therapy. The guideline is produced via the Protocol Authoring tools developed in Prestige. The output can then be handled by the Protocol Manager and produce recommendations to clinicians across the health care system.

A.7.3.2 Neurology

The main objective of the Neurology Scenario is to use information technology to support the implementation of protocol directed shared care for the management of epilepsy between general practices and specialist centres. Hospital Egas Moniz (HEM), Lisbon acts as a specialist centre, and Centro Saúde da Ajuda (CSA) is the primary care centre, involved in the project, from which patients are referred to HEM.

Gentofte Hospital in Copenhagen is developing multimedia neurology teleconsultation services, also with a focus on epilepsy including the implementation of a specialised database for neurophysiology (e.g. electro-encephalography) departments.

A.7.3.3 Diabetes

The Diabetes sub-project in *PRESTIGE* addresses the implementation of a guideline application concerning the diagnosis and management of Non-Insulin Dependant (Type II) Diabetes Mellitus, focusing on primary care management by general practitioners and practice nurses/ nurse practitioners and support for patient self-management, with referral to specialist centres.

This pilot diabetes mellitus guideline application is mainly targeted to use at Long Eaton Health Centre, Nottingham (Trent region, UK) and, then at Centro Saúde Ajuda, Health Region of Lisboa and Tejo Valley, PT.

A.7.3.4 Primary care

Primary Health care is the largest sub project in *PRESTIGE*, reflecting the advanced state of informatics in this sector in several countries, and the active interest in guideline development and telematics R&D within the user communities, as represented in the *PRESTIGE* consortium. This strong platform in the primary sector provides a favourable basis for the wider development of protocol-assisted health telematics across the community/hospital interface.

The Primary Care Sub-Project in *PRESTIGE* is split into three clinical scenarios according to the distinct countries / health regions involved, namely A) Netherlands, B) Emilia Romagna Region, IT and C) UK.

A.7.3.4.1 Netherlands

In the Netherlands, the Dutch College of General Practitioners (NHG is an Associated Partner in *PRESTIGE*) is responsible for the development of guidelines for care in general practice. Over 50 of those guidelines ("standards of care", or "NHG standards") have been published. The guidelines are based on consensus, reached by a panel of experts, and are well accepted by Dutch GPs, as well as by patients.

NHG-developed guidelines for influenza vaccination and cervical screening are being implemented using the *PRESTIGE* tools. Both types of population directed care result from agreements between the Dutch ministry of Health and the Dutch Association of General Practitioners (LHV). LHV and NHG together have set up an organisation to support the introduction and execution of the preventative activities.

A.7.3.4.2 Emilia Romagna Region, Modena Local Health Unit

Target healthcare activities in Modena Local Health Unit, Emilia Romagna Region, include primary care management by general practitioners with a focus on the locally adapted guidelines for influenza vaccination and cervical cancer screening. This local guideline implementation activities are being undertaken in co-operation with SIMG (Società Italiana di Medicina Generale), also involved in *PRESTIGE*, and which is concerned with the professional development and information dissemination about clinical guidelines and informatic tools in medicine.

There is also a convergence of the objectives of *PRESTIGE* with the plans of the Regional Health Authority in the Emilia Romagna Region for the creation of an integrated Regional Health Care System.

A.7.3.4.3 UK

The major interface activities in the UK are grouped within the Cardiology and Diabetes sub projects, described above, which are implementing primary care guidelines for diabetes management and angina. In addition, the Sowerby Unit, Northern Region, have worked closely with the North of England Guideline Development Group based at the Centre for Health Services Research in Newcastle University. In March 1996 the North of England Evidence based Asthma Guideline was published both in the British Medical Journal and in full on the world wide web. At the Sowerby Unit the implementation of this gold-standard guideline has been adapted for computerised implementation concerning Asthma Diagnosis and Management.

A.7.4 RHCN services provided by the project

As above described, *PRESTIGE* aims at providing a telematic infra-structure enabling the implementation and dissemination of computerised guidelines in both primary care and hospital settings, in each case addressing problems of co-operative and shared care between these sectors. The services provided are based on an unified set of generic technology components which can be used in all telematics applications for implementing clinical guidelines, and comprising:

- The conceptual basis of the *PRESTIGE* environment is featured by two complementary important pieces. They together provide a single reference schema for the integration of the various servers and ensure the internal consistency of the whole system:
  - the conceptual model
  - the architecture of the *PRESTIGE* environment. Starting from the requirements of the *PRESTIGE* environment user, it provides a continuum from the description of the user interactions with the system, up to the design of the software components which together implement the functionality.
- A series of software components, which conform to the design above, and their implementation as servers operating in a client-server environment. Generally speaking, each server encapsulates its own databases and provides to its clients a certain number of services which can be activated through a set of API

functions. Examples of such servers are: Act Manager and Protocol Manager, Electronic Patient Record Manager, Enterprise Manager.

- A set of knowledge management facilities that protocol processing invokes at run-time. This environment offers two subsets of such facilities:
  - semantic management which allows to represent and exploit the semantics of the domain. It is mainly used for the structuring and retrieval of medical information in the Electronic Patient Record.
  - inference management and temporal constraints management. It is mainly used by the protocol engine when processing protocols.

- Protocol authoring facilities through the provision of a dedicated tool, entitled Guideline Authoring and Dissemination Tool (GAUDI), relying on a set of terminology services. This is an off-line service which allows to input and update protocols which are then exported to the run-time environment through a suitable interchange format.

- Semantic model configuration facilities through the provision of a dedicated tool implemented by using the Internet/Web technology. This is an off-line service which allows to populate the SeM knowledge base.

The *PRESTIGE* Conceptual Model represents the basis of the telematics applications for clinical guideline implementation in the project. Specifically, it is the source for the engineering development of the *PRESTIGE* generic technology components which have been produced. The Model has two major subdivisions. The first describes healthcare in general, and the second focuses on clinical protocols.

The Conceptual Model is intended to provide a conceptual basis for all generic, application-related software engineering in the project, thereby ensuring full conceptual coherence across the component set. Particular attention has been paid to modelling the:

- *healthcare enterprise*, thought of as the generic enterprise encompassing primary and secondary care;

- *authorisation and access*, as there are risks & constraints associated with any access to patient information,

- *knowledge*, as guideline applications are knowledge-based applications. Guidelines are modules of clinical knowledge and the function of telematics guideline applications are to assist the availability, accessibility and appropriate use of that knowledge. This requires an explicit model defining standard formats for computerised representation and use of items of knowledge.

- *act management*, viewing acts as units of activity which when properly modelled and implemented are able to support the orderly planning and execution of clinical work, and the proper co-ordination of work between co-operating clinicians.

- *protocols*, as the *PRESTIGE* Protocol Model provides rules defining the knowledge statement constructs which can appear in a *PRESTIGE* protocol knowledge base. As an Object model, it defines the kinds of entities (objects) which may appear in the protocol, with their permitted relations and attributes. Several main types of these objects can be identified:

- general *concepts* (acts and case-specific phenomena such as diagnoses and symptoms);
- overall protocol and its component parts (all *individual, named instances* of the concept PROTOCOL);
- *expressions*, built out of concepts, instance names and syntax operations. They can be used in *conditions* governing the appropriate use of a protocol or its parts or *methods* defining specific attribute values.
- *templates* which define a set of data items which are to be collected.

- *patient data,* as telematics support for clinical guidelines needs not only knowledge bases and knowledge models, but a mature electronic patient record (EPR). Clinical guidelines define patient-specific recommendations where the option selected is a function of the patient's medical condition and other factors which is obtained by directly interrogating the patient record. Moreover a record should be capable of keeping track of how a guideline is used over time, since later options are also determined, amongst other things, by choices made earlier. An important part of the *PRESTIGE* model is therefore the patient record which defines what kinds of information a *PRESTIGE* application EPR must be able to represent.

Together with the *PRESTIGE* Conceptual Model, an open architecture for interoperability supporting the design and exploitation of clinical guidelines has been defined. The *PRESTIGE* Architecture specifies the external behaviour of the *PRESTIGE* system components, but not their internal characteristics. On the contrary it defines system components as objects, encapsulations of data and functions, providing services to other objects and using other objects' services. The external behaviour of these system components is fully described by the addition of the description of the constraints between objects' services.

The components of the *PRESTIGE* Architecture are shown in Figure D.16 below. The numbered circles represent Service Access Points - the generic open interfaces between *PRESTIGE* and/or legacy system technology components

The *PRESTIGE* architectural framework is based on the following relevant standards:
- ISO/ICE/TIC/SC21/WG7 – Basic Reference Model for Open Distributed Processing
- CEN TC251/ N95-261 – Healthcare Information Framework
- CEN TC251/ N95-285 – Standard Architecture for Healthcare Information Systems
- CEN TC251/PrENV 12265 – Electronic Health Care Record Architecture
- European pre-standard for healthcare information systems – the RICHE Reference Architecture

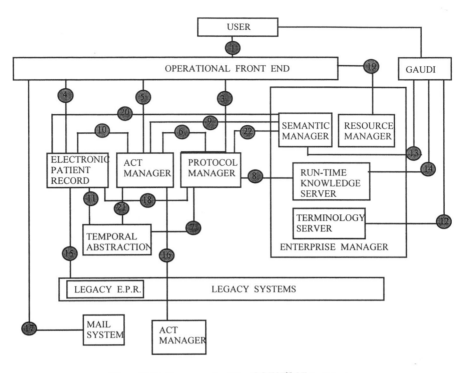

Figure D.16: Components of the *PRESTIGE* Architecture

The architectural specifications provide a mapping between user expectations and system developers design. They cover only the scope of the *PRESTIGE* project, that is the management of clinical guidelines, and do not describe other areas like the management of acts or the management of clinical data or electronic healthcare records. In order to design a system able to manage clinical guidelines and to insert this system within a global architectural framework such as the European pre-standard HISA, the services provided by system components also able to support other areas have been used. The architectural specifications do not pretend to fully specify the services such system components should provide when they are used outside of the *PRESTIGE* scope.

The interfaces between system components as they are described represent *PRESTIGE* *PRESTIGE* needs in terms of services and parameters. When suppliers develop such system components they have to take into account criteria linked to performance aspects and technologies available and also take into account the services such component should provide also for other domain areas than the management and support of clinical guidelines. Therefore some of the interface definitions may be refined into for example more granular services at the implementation time.

The way applications can use these services is described below.

A.7.5 RHCN technical systems used in the project

The objectives of the generic technologies above introduced have been to design and develop the architectural and technological environment on top of which the *PRESTIGE* functionality can be implemented and operated taking into account the great diversity of legacy environments, particular needs and situations shown by the consortium. This approach enabled the project to deliver a truly generic approach in terms of architecture and software components which can then be implemented and operated in a variety of sites.

Therefore, each application site should integrate the generic technologies with their own legacy systems by means of the services offered by the *PRESTIGE* system, such as:

- The *PRESTIGE* Protocol Manager (PPM) is supplied as framework of C++ classes derived from the Conceptual Model that may be embedded in an application to provide protocol-directed recommendations about acts to be performed with regard to a subject. The protocol manager has been implemented as a class hierarchy and have two software interfaces. An application interface that is the mechanism by which applications access protocol management functions and receive any returned information. All applications must comply with this interface. The virtual interface allows the protocol manager to access the EPR, Act Manager, and run-time knowledge. All implementations of *PRESTIGE* architecture must comply with this interface.

- A *PRESTIGE* application requires an Electronic Patient Record satisfying specified generic properties. A generic implementation of a *PRESTIGE* EPR has been created and is available in a form which operated on UNIX platforms, suitable for use in conjunction with the Act Management module. *PRESTIGE* applications have the option, where their local requirements and legacy technology make this preferable, of creating or adapting a local EPR to comply with the *PRESTIGE* specification.

- Protocols are authored using a constrained terminology and a tool known as the GAUDI (Guideline AUthoring and DIssemination tool). The GAUDI formalises paper or template representations of protocols and translates them into a form that can be used at run time, as stored in the Run-Time Knowledge Server (see below). The constrained terminology ensures that the Protocol Manager, when working with a run-time version of a guideline, understands the terms it reads from the Electronic Patient Record and can relate those terms to those contained in the Run-Time Knowledge Server.

- The form in which protocols are represented electronically in *PRESTIGE* applications is specified in the *PRESTIGE* Conceptual Model, from which is derived a BNF grammar specification of the protocol knowledge which may be entered into and exported from the *PRESTIGE* Protocol Authoring Tool (GAUDI). Within the *PRESTIGE* Run Time system, the information requirements to be provided for the Protocol Manager by the Knowledge Server are contained in the specification of the Protocol Manager's interface requirements. The specification takes the form of a set of abstract C++ functions with their associated class definitions. Each *PRESTIGE* application is responsible for the concrete implementation of its Knowledge server using the database platform appropriate to that application.

- A generic Act Manager has been build as part of the suite of generic server provided by *PRESTIGE*. This provides facilities to control and manage the performing and recording of healthcare acts and their results. The technology is designed to support multiple communicating Act Managers linked to distributed departmental systems which are capable of supporting co-operative professional work by managing the information flows involved in acts (such as a blood test) which may be requested by one department and performed by another.

Each application site is responsible for their communication facilities.

Requirements for security for all technology developed at *PRESTIGE* are taken from the CEN document Medical Informatics Secure User Identification for Health Care: Management and Security of Passwords - Health Care Oriented IT Security Functionality Class.

A.7.6 RHCN products resulting from the project

A.7.6.1 Business opportunities

Clinical practice guidelines may be defined as 'systematically developed statements to assist practitioner and patient decisions about appropriate health care for specific clinical circumstances'. Governmental institutions, national medical initiatives and the scientific community have achieved a large consensus in the past few years regarding the value of clinical practice guidelines, criteria for the development of sound guidelines, and the conditions of their effective dissemination and implementation.

The use of clinical guidelines and use of telematics tools to aid this process will be an important instrument for attaining government and purchaser objectives in terms of cost-effective health care, and may become an obligatory element in future service contracts. Consequently, a large new added-value market for such products is expected in many areas of existing health telematics business.

The primary care market is maturing rapidly in a number of European countries. In the UK and Netherlands most GPs use a computer for aspects of patient management, and the majority will soon use a computer for medical records. The addition of protocol tools to GP commercial practice systems can enhance the value and competitive appeal of these products. This is clearly illustrated by means of several commercial partners in the primary care sector participating in *PRESTIGE* (AAH Meditel Ltd (United Kingdom), THETA (Italy), Cendata (The Netherlands), Rambøll (Denmark)), which are now developing enhanced forms of their existing products incorporating telematics for guideline support integrated during *PRESTIGE*.

The development of patient-centred information systems and electronic patient records in hospital has been, on the whole, relatively slow. *PRESTIGE* can work as a catalyst to develop this market, through the incentives of support for co-operative care and protocol-directed care. The strong basis of *PRESTIGE* in the primary care sector provides a sound footing for primary/secondary co-operative care systems which will further open up new markets for hospital-based telematics. Several commercial and health service partners in *PRESTIGE* (SNI, OSE, Saphis, NHS IMC) view *PRESTIGE* as providing a logical extension to the emerging HIS systems integration standards issuing from the work of

RICHE and NUCLEUS to exploit the added-value potential of services for protocol-directed care management.

A.7.6.2 End products of the project

Key end products of *PRESTIGE* include:

- The *PRESTIGE* **Reference Model**, comprising the *PRESTIGE* Conceptual Model and related Architecture, enables healthcare telematics application developers and users to use a public model for electronic guideline knowledge representation allowing 'plug and play' integration of published electronic guidelines across European healthcare sites. Through the public APIs delivered interoperability of generic *PRESTIGE* components with existing application infrastructure is enabled.

- **GAUDI**: Guideline Authoring and Dissemination Tool, supports electronic knowledge authoring of clinical guideline by central clinical bodies and local guideline tailoring by clinical end-users. Ensures built-in compliance of knowledge bases with a common knowledge model, ensuring transferability and interoperability in healthcare applications.

- *PRESTIGE* Runtime generic Components including Protocol Manager, Act Manager, Electronic Patient Record, Knowledge Management Server and the Enterprise Manager. These components provide telematics support for implementation of clinical guidelines and protocols. Application vendors may link selected components in platform-specific versions to existing legacy system infrastructure.

- *PRESTIGE* telematics dissemination resources for clinical guidelines and protocols, comprising tools, materials and services, providing a coherent set of solutions for clinical guideline dissemination and implementation, while decentralising open access by European clinicians and citizens to information and evidence on best practice.

- *PRESTIGE* Application Sub-projects, which will report their validation results and identify key success factors in the use of *PRESTIGE* tools. Each application is expected to become a permanent, sustainable part of local clinical practice support.

A.7.7 Lessons learnt from project

Clinical practice guidelines have emerged as a major strategy to improve quality and efficiency in health services by optimising the practical application of evidence deriving from rigorous research. The *PRESTIGE* project has created and implemented a strategy focusing health telematics services around support for clinical guideline dissemination and implementation. Because the clinical guideline movement is firmly based within the clinical and health service policy communities, this focus guarantees a strongly user-driven agenda for technology procurement. Because of its close linkage to goals defined within the user community, it helps ensure that the potential of technology will be effectively exploited.

Clinical practice guidelines define not only best clinical practice but best organisational practice for co-operative healthcare; implementing such guidelines therefore creates intensive new demands on the set of telematics services needed to support healthcare organisation, i.e. regional healthcare networks (RHCN).

A significant unforeseen factor has been the amount of effort required in almost all project's applications to define, refine or adapt the clinical guidelines selected for implementation in a sufficiently precise and appropriate form for local implementation supported by telematics. The benefit from this additional required effort has been the creation of a European community of expertise in the definition and representation of this increasingly important category of healthcare information. At the same time the project has translated this experience into tools and methods which can be shared in the future by European bodies concerned with creation and dissemination of guidelines.

The adherence to a sound generic development strategy has enabled a common application integration approach to be used in the different organisational and technical environments of the project's different application sites, based on a common understanding and common design concepts. However, the project had to face a considerable, and sometimes difficult, learning curve in achieving shared understanding of such new design and functional concepts, which could be, translated into practical development plans in widely varying local situations.

Despite those difficulties all the project's applications are implementing real guideline applications with a sure future in terms of industrial and healthcare exploitation. Specific plans for exploiting *PRESTIGE* results through leading national products for Hospital Information Systems and GP practice systems exist or are being formulated in France, Portugal, the Netherlands, Denmark, Italy and the UK. The commercial partners' practical commitments to integrating project products into their legacy systems provides the most convincing endorsement of the generality and interoperability of the *PRESTIGE* concepts.

A.8. REMEDES

A.8.1 *Purpose of the project*

The project is aimed at developing and implementing a set of telematic services encompassing the bulk of the information exchange between primary and secondary care.

The main challenge of the project is to demonstrate that there are sufficient common elements between one health care system and another to justify a central design of the solution and the constitution of a single library of configurable objects. The health care systems include those based on both a liberal medicine model, and also on a public, structured system.

A.8.2 *Regions participating in the project in general*

REMEDES has pilot sites in four different European countries: France, Italy, Spain and the UK. The Regions are described below.

A.8.2.1 Montpellier

The pilot site in France is the area comprised in the Montpellier District in the Languedoc-Roussillon region of Southern France. Montpellier is a provincial capital and the home of the oldest medicine school in Europe. The District covers the town and the surrounding rural area with a total population of 300.000.

The area is particularly well served in terms of health care with one of the largest public teaching hospitals in the whole country and 13 private clinics offering a total of over 4.000 beds. 478 GPs practice in the area within a context of liberal medicine.

The local partners of REMEDES are:

- Technopole Montpellier/Languedoc/Roussillon, the local Development Agency, acting as co-ordinator for the pilot site;

- OLSY France, the technical partner, which belongs to the same group of companies as the overall REMEDES co-ordinator Olivetti Sanità;

- CHU de Montpellier, the local public teaching hospital, which is ranked 5th in size among all the French hospitals of this kind. Moreover the CHU is the largest single employer in the Languedoc-Roussillon region with staff in excess of 9.000, 1.500 of which are physicians;

- Union Professionelle des Medécins Libéraux, the official body which represents all the medical doctors practising as independent professionals in the region (roughly 5.500);

- Chambre Syndicale des Pharmaciens, the representative body of pharmacists, with about 280 members out of the 380 pharmacists practising in the region.

There are talks underway with Languedoc Mutualité and several private clinics for them to participate in the validation activities in Montpellier.

A.8.2.2 Regione Lombardia - Bergamo

This Italian pilot site in located in the north-eastern section of Lombardy around the provincial capital of Bergamo, a medium-seized industrial town. The area for which the ASL (Ambito Sanitario Locale) has to provide Health Care shows a good spectrum of settings, varying from the urban town centre to sparse population in the mountain area of the Alps. The total population covered is about 380.000, who are looked after by 327 GPs and 29 Free-Choice Paediatricians, distributed over 15 Health Districts.

The Secondary Care infrastructure comprises four public hospitals with a total of 2.150 beds, and five smaller private clinics.

The local partners of REMEDES are:

- ASL 12 di Bergamo, the Local Health Authority;

- SIMG (Società Italiana di Medicina Generale) the Italian scientific association of General Practitioners;

- Olivetti Sanità, Co-ordinating Contractor of REMEDES and, together with Sema Group, the main industrial partner in the Consortium;

- Datasoft Management, an independent software supplier from Belgium, providing the EHCR environment for GPs.

A.8.2.3 Regione Lombardia - Melegnano

This is a small satellite town located in the south-eastern area of Greater Milan in Italy. The local population is 150.000, who are looked after by a total of 140 Primary Care professionals among GPs and Free-Choice Paediatricians distributed over five Health Districts. The area is a mixture of urban and rural settings, but communications between one and the other are good because of the favourable nature of the local geography (the Po valley).

The Secondary Care infrastructure comprises one public hospital and one large private clinic.

The local partners of REMEDES are:

- ASL 26 di Melegnano, the Local Health Authority;

- Olivetti Sanità, Co-ordinating Contractor of REMEDES and, together with Sema Group, the main industrial partner in the Consortium;

- Datasoft Management, an independent software supplier from Belgium, providing the EHCR environment for GPs.

The validation in Melegnano is totally funded by the local partners of REMEDES without any contribution from the EU.

A.8.2.4 Cambridge and Huntingdon

Cambridge and Huntingdon Health Authority is a district health authority, part of the NHS in the UK, covering a population of 420.000 in East Anglia region of England with an annual budget of £200m. The area is rural in nature, but with a few large cities. The Health Authority purchases services principally from four hospitals, about 200 GPs organised in 60 group practices, and two community units.

The local partners of REMEDES are:

- Cambridge and Huntingdon Health Authority, the Local Health Authority.

- Sema Group UK, the British arm of the Anglo-French consultancy, system integration and outsourcing provider, acting as technical partner.

- Addenbrooke's Hospital is a major teaching hospital within the Cambridge and Huntingdon area. The hospital has about 1,000 beds, and has strong research links with Cambridge University and the Medical Research Council. As well as being a district hospital and teaching hospital, it is regarded as a tertiary referral centre for the area for cancer care. The Trust also has two smaller hospitals, and employs some 5.000 staff.

- Local GPs.

A.8.2.5 Comunidad Autónoma de Madrid – Arca de Salud VIII

Health Area VIII is located in the south-western part of the Madrid Autonomous Community. The geographical characteristics of this area are those of a transitional zone between an urban or metropolitan area with satellite cities like Móstoles and Alcorcón, and a rural zone whose most important town is Navalcarnero.

Health Area VIII is made up of 19 municipalities grouped into three health districts: two urban districts corresponding to Móstoles and Alcorcón, and one rural district in Navalcarnero. Each district is subdivided into smaller entities called basic zones.

The local population is about 400.000, of which 52% lives in Móstoles, 30% in Alcorcón and 9% in Navalcarnero.

The area is served by 20 Primary Care Centres and by two public hospitals, one of which is brand-new, with a total capacity of over 1.000 beds. The medical staff is composed of 247 GPs and 270 specialists.

The local partners of REMEDES are:

- Hospital General de Móstoles.

- Sema Group Spain, the Spanish arm of the Anglo-French consultancy, system integration and outsourcing provider, acting as technical partner.

A.8.2.6 Baleares – Manacor

The town of Manacor (25.500 inhabitants) is located in the south-eastern portion of the Mallorca island. From a health care point of view, Manacor is the centre of an area comprising 20 smaller towns and villages with a total population of 108.270. Due to its geographical situation (a fair number of villages not belonging to the Health Area are nearer to Manacor than to the capital Palma) the catchment area of Manacor is in reality as large as 145.000.

The geographical and socio-economic characteristics of the area can be summarised as follows:

- mature population with a moderate growth rate (3,4% between 1986-1991);

- increasing incidence of the over-65 age group (19,2% as opposed to 14,6% in the rest of the Island);

- strong growth of the population during the summer period (up to 50%);

- good socio-economic context with a well-developed service sector;

- poor transportation infrastructure (despite short distances, travelling time to Manacor from surrounding towns can take up to an hour).

The area is served by nine Primary Care Centres and by a brand-new public hospital, with a capacity of over 191 beds. The medical staff is composed of 90 GPs and 77 specialists.

The local partners of REMEDES are:

- Hospital Fundación de Manacor;
- Sema Group Spain, acting as technical partner.

Manacor is not yet officially recognised as a pilot site of REMEDES, although the procedure for its inclusion has been initiated.

A.8.3 Regional partners in the RHCN build by the project

Apart the partners already mentioned in relation to individual pilot sites, two more partners, both having the status of full Contractors, complete the Consortium set-up. Within the Consortium these partners have a role which spans across the various pilot site.

CHC is a consortium that groups hospitals and health care centres and whose members are Local Authorities and non-profit Foundations in the Catalonia region. It comprises 45 hospitals and health care centres providing a total of 5.500 beds for acute treatment and 1.100 long-stay beds and employs over 10.000 staff. CHC represents roughly 35% of the health care infrastructure in Catalonia CHC collaborates on the definition of the evaluation criteria for the validation phase and in the organisation of the Spanish user group.

MediBRIDGE is an organisation offering first-generation telematics services in Belgium The service has currently more than 3.500 "medical mail boxes"; and the customer base is still growing. The services are presently offered to health care professionals such as community pharmacists and paramedical staff. MediBRIDGE has collaborated with Datasoft Management for the message definition, the message builder(s) development. It has also collaborated in the definition of the services through its expertise in setting up and commercialising telematic services in Belgium.

A.8.4 RHCN services provided by the project

Laboratory test Request & Results Reporting: This service is used when the GP is able to take the required sample from the patient and has to send it to a laboratory which will be carrying out the tests. The service will enable advance notification of the test to the laboratory. This notification can include patient details, details of requested tests and any special instructions or comments. The test results will be returned electronically to the health professional requesting the test, and can be incorporated automatically into the local system.

Diagnostic procedure Request & Results Reporting: This service is used when the patient has to attend a special centre for a diagnostic procedure, which the GP can not perform himself. This service enables the GP to select the most suitable clinic with the patient, and book the patient into the clinic of his choice. A Clinic Centre List will identify all clinics able to carry out the test. The information transmitted with the request can include patient details, details of requested tests and any special instructions or comments. The test results will be returned electronically to the health professional requesting the test, and can be incorporated automatically into the local system. While the results can incorporate images these would normally not be used by the GP for diagnostic purposes.

Referral/Outpatient Booking: This service is used when the patient needs a consultation with a specialist for his medical condition. The service enables the GP to access the outpatient booking system, and agree a suitable time with the patient. Patient details and GP comments are automatically transferred to the outpatient system to initiate the relevant computer and clerical activities within the outpatient department. The appointment details will be transferred to the patient record on the practice computer and a hard copy will be printed for the patient. The actual booking and confirmation can be carried out by administrative staff. If Medical Conferencing facilities are available they can be used, where appropriate to make a visual image to attach to the referral. The visual image can also be annotated by the GP through white-board type facilities. The results of the consultation will be returned electronically to the health professional requesting the referral, and can be incorporated directly into the local system.

Hospitalisation Request: The hospitalisation request, currently a paper document given to the patient, will be forwarded electronically to the hospital, using if possible standard coding for medical data. The selection of the preferred hospital will be supported by an enquiry facility on the waiting lists of the various clinical departments in different hospitals. In addition, the GP can extract from his own medical records database a summary of the medical history of the patient and attach it to the request for hospitalisation; this would include the results of the tests carried out prior to admission, and which were used in arriving at the decision to admit. Medical Database Enquiry service can be used in conjunction with this, to communicate pre-admission protocols to GPs. This will ensure all necessary procedures/investigations are carried out prior to admission.

Hospital Discharge Summary: After an episode of hospital care, whether in-patient or day-care, a summary of the episode will be sent by the hospital to the GP. Details should include diagnosis, treatment and outcome, and details of drugs supplied to the patient on discharge.

Clinical Balance during Therapy (Shared Care): After a period of hospitalisation, or referral to a specialist clinic, either for surgical operations or other treatments, there could be a need for a follow-up treatment, possibly rehabilitation or continuing course of drugs. The GP who monitors the evolution of the patient's condition, transmits to the relevant service/department of the hospital the post follow-up clinical balance of the patient; this avoids the use of the patient himself as a carrier of information. The GP can equally have access to the service/department above during the follow-up treatment for consulting with the specialist who treated the patient. The service support shared care arrangements, both when the hospital retains responsibility for treatment after a patient has returned home, and when responsibility transfers to the GP.

Medical Statistics Reporting: This service will handle large volumes of patient identifiable data such as diagnosis, referrals, tests, procedures and outcomes. This data, after it has been anonymised, will become part of an important information database. The numerous sources for data collection and the several different techniques that are possible in enhancing the usefulness of this data make the provision of this service of great assistance to all health planners and those charged with the safe, cost effective management of health care services. GPs can use this service to evaluate their clinical activity by comparing with others, and to identify opportunities to improve the service they offer to their patients.

Value Added Services: Next to the Primary Services described above, a number of Value Added Services are provided, which vary from Primary Service to Primary Service, but include some or all of the following:
  • reminders of outstanding clinical service requests;
  • checklists (paper or electronic) of services provided to either initiate or check the invoicing for the services;
  • analysis of elapsed time between requests for clinical services, and completion of the service;
  • comparative analysis of services requested;
  • provide (anonymous) data for epidemiological analysis, for example by geographic area, against demographic markers, etc.
  • comparative analysis between service providers.

A.8.5 RHCN technical systems used in the project

REMEDES Services

Some of the REMEDES services are on-line access (client server), some of them batch access (store and forward) using mail clients, and some a mixture of the two types of access. REMEDES also requires on-line access to the secondary care systems for the on-line booking services.

Components of the REMEDES service

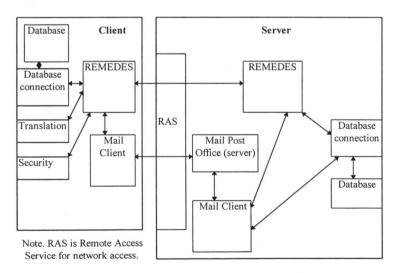

Figure D.17: Components of the REMEDES Service

Figure D.17 shows the generic component parts of the REMEDES service. The REMEDES software does not have to physically reside on the server or the client. It can be either dynamically configured or permanently configured as the need arises. Indeed the

REMEDES application can be run on a separate server and the REMEDES client can be configured as a server on a local area network. The database shown for the client can reside on the server or on the client.

The following table describes the components in the component diagram.

Table D.1: Description of REMEDES Components

Component	Description
REMEDES CLIENT	
Translation	Translate to and from GP system format, this can be proprietary or a standard such as EDIFACT
Security	The encryption of sensitive data, authentication and digital signature
Mail Client	The sending and receipt of messages
REMEDES	Functions to use the REMEDES service, link to the communications and existing systems
Database	An SQL compliant database connected using JDBC driver, contains details of items of services used, configuration etc.
REMEDES SERVER	
Remote Access Service	Controls the log-on, user configuration etc. of remote clients.
Mail Post Office	Routing mail messages
Mail Client	Receipt and sending of messages to and from the REMEDES system e.g. error messages
REMEDES	Functionality to provide security, re-routing, user statistics, medical statistics, on-line booking etc.
Database	An SQL database to store Information for medical statistics, logging and audit trails, selection of appointments etc.
Database connection	Access to the database in a standard way

The REMEDES system is built from existing components where it is both cost effective and feasible to do so. The choice of components is also influenced by the need to future proof the applications as far as possible.

The REMEDES system is designed to allow the use of components from alternative sources, thus not restricting the future implementations of the service in alternative environments. For instance the use of Microsoft's Access database for a local database does not preclude the use of other SQL compatible databases located on any accessible server.

The REMEDES server software also maintains portability to UNIX.

Selected software components

The following software components have been identified for use with REMEDES:

Table D.2: REMEDES Software Components

Components	Product/Supplier
Server Operating System	Windows NT Microsoft Information server version 4.0
Client Operating System	Windows 95 for the pilot implementation
Server Database	Oracle 7 (see note 1)
Client Database	Access (see note 1)
Store and forward (e-mail)	Microsoft Exchange version 5 Note it is necessary to have the full Exchange server not just the work group exchange mail
Client server	Windows NT & Microsoft Remote Access Services (RAS)
Development language	Java version 1.1 (see note 2)
HTML Viewer	Microsoft Internet Explorer (part of Win NT & 95) and distributed free of charge
Translation	EDIFACT - Prospera (Visual EDI & Vedi/x)
Encryption	PGP, however if required it will conform to national rules and practices.
Authentication	Strong authentication will be used for dial up access in the UK, otherwise it will depend upon national rules and practices.
Digital signature	Not chosen yet. It will depend upon national rules and practices.
Automated scripting tools. These may be required as part of bridging software, which is outside of the scope of the REMEDES development, however required for the project implementation	Citation Link1000 Microscribe knowledgeware flashpoint Web View (Olivetti)
Communications systems Management	System Management Server (SMS, Microsoft for Win' NT)

Note 1. This should be an SQL compliant database, so that alternative databases can be used if required.

Note 2. The performance of Java software will be evaluated during the development and if required C++ and DBMS features will be used for performance reasons.

Figure D.18 shows the chosen components in place.

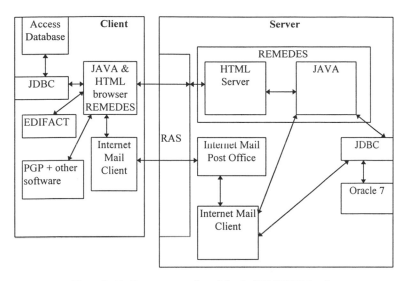

Figure D.18: Components selected for the REMEDES Service

A.8.6 RHCN products resulting from the project

The intention of REMEDES, from its inception, has always been to produce a Demonstrator of industrial quality, which could be used subsequently for the commercial provision of services.

Business opportunities vary very much from one country to the other, with the UK clearly lying at the bottom of the scale, and with Italy offering the brightest future. France constitutes for the time being the biggest question mark, because the addition of Montpellier to the list of pilot site is very recent and because the business case of REMEDES (… or of any telematic service) is more difficult to define.

The two main industrial partners, Olivetti Sanità and Sema Group, have already started the commercial activities around REMEDES and a number of offers have already been produced in Italy and in Spain. There are also reasonable chances of a new company being created in Italy to commercialise there the EHCR products by Datasoft Management, which are now fully integrated in the REMEDES Service.

A.8.7 Lessons learnt from project

During the life of the REMEDES project a number of problems have been encountered:

Long life cycle

This is a problem totally related to the internal management of the project. Too much time has gone by between the moment the REMEDES concepts were defined and the time the first release of the Demonstrator was ready to be shipped. This problem, today to a great extent solved, has led to frustration both inside the development team and among the potential users.

Some justifications can be drawn from the somewhat over-ambitious targets that the Consortium has fixed for itself:

- central design of the Demonstrator;
- single implementation of the Demonstrator for all the countries;
- development work split between two different teams and locations sharing a common development environment and Object Model;
- use of modern development methodology unfamiliar to the development team;
- industrial quality of the Demonstrator.

Insufficient penetration of standards

The need for a telematic service, such as REMEDES, to link into a variety of end systems to exchange data or to give interactive access to appointment facilities, makes life extremely difficult in the absence of recognised and widespread standards.

In most of the areas addressed by REMEDES, European EDIFACT standards do exist but their national implementation is still lacking (this is the reason the CoCo project has a strong justification).

In the absence of standards, REMEDES and its brother projects need to adapt to every change in the end systems, the evolution of which is beyond the control of the telematic service provider. This can be costly and inefficient, with a risk of disruption to the service because of de-synchronisation between the telematic service and the systems it has to talk to.

Change in the Health Care context

The reality of RHCN today is that they are still and too often the initiative of one or more enlightened persons who see in them an indispensable tool for health care delivery, rationalisation and improved quality. This means that when people change job, sometimes the interest in a RHCN project vanishes, because it did not represent a corporate commitment.

Even when RHCN correspond to a corporate commitment by the national health system, there is no guarantee that the commitment will last long enough, or receive the support needed at grass roots level, for the project to be fully implemented: health networks were the flavour of the month in the UK when REMEDES started, but although the national commitment to them has been restated recently, at local level there are often other priorities.

Sometimes the organisation of a national health system can evolve in a direction which can affect positively or negatively the appeal of a given telematic service: the appeal of the REMEDES on-line booking service has been boosted in Lombardy, where, through consolidation of Health Authorities, a single ASL has to offer a single and consistent interface to heterogeneous appointment systems it has inherited from its predecessors.

A.9. Star

A.9.1 Purpose

Care for patients is increasingly being delivered by different specialists in different locations - acute hospitals, community hospitals, general practice surgeries or in the home. This leads to greater demands on the administration and management of patient-related information, both within the organisation and between organisations. The traditional method of transferring information about a patient was with a paper document - a referral letter, discharge letter or report - and whilst in a hospital, case notes physically followed the patient between different departments. As hospitals and other healthcare institutions have become computerised, patient data is captured in each department and the medical record is available at all times anywhere within the unit.

Unfortunately there is still a gap when it comes to communicating between different healthcare institutions and information still 'flows' on paper, fax or by telephone. With the increased use of specialist care and with the 'commercial' pressures to increase the flow of patients through the healthcare system, there is a clear requirement to replace the paper-based communication with something more efficient. This not only requires the telecommunications infrastructure but also agreement on medical record standards, security and confidentiality, support for co-operative working to enable healthcare professionals to give advice to colleagues in distant locations, and the optimal use of resources across organisational boundaries.

Star☆ has selected key regions across Europe at which the benefits will be demonstrated of sharing healthcare information between one or more hospitals and their surrounding healthcare providers. The complementary results of previous EU projects are brought together to form a common set of proven solutions for European healthcare. Using basic middleware services, end-user applications across a region are able to share parts of the medical record, make rational decisions on planning whole episodes of care (not just interventions), schedule other healthcare functions via an interactive referral process, make more informed management decisions about resources, and provide the building blocks for co-operative diagnosis and treatment.

A.9.2 Regions participating in the project in general

A.9.2.1 North Eastern Health Board

NEHB is located in the north eastern region of the Republic of Ireland and comprises the counties of Cavan, Monaghan, Meath and Louth, and has a population of 302.000. NEHB will be working closely with their sister board, the North Western Health Board, which is located to the north west of the island, and covers the counties of Donegal, Leitrim and Sligo, with a population of 208.000. These Boards are two of Ireland's eight regional Health Boards. Each Board administers services in its area and is responsible for both hospital, community and primary care sectors

A.9.2.2 Stockholm

Huddinge University Hospital is one of two major research and teaching hospitals in the Stockholm area. Clinically oriented research is abundant throughout the organisation.

Many of the 38 Clinical Departments and Diagnostic Laboratories have attained international prominence.

Huddinge University Hospital is one of ten major regional hospitals in Sweden. It provides a full range of medical services. Medical care is given to approximately 45.000 inpatients annually; there are more than 580.000 outpatient visits, of which 370.000 are with physicians. The basic catchment area has a population of 250.000. The hospital has 1.200 beds including geriatric and psychiatric beds. Patients are also referred from the greater Stockholm area, from other parts of Sweden, and from abroad.

The hospital is affiliated with the Karolinska Institute Medical University. Several categories of students in the medical and related fields receive parts of their education at Huddinge. There are high school students, orderlies, nursing attendants, as well as medical students, nurse students and others. Annually, 1.000 medical students are taught in various courses at the hospital. In addition, tuition and training of physicians at various levels of their basic and specialist training is performed.

Huddinge University Hospital has its primary catchment area in the southern parts of Stockholm. In that area, a working relationship has been long established with Södertälje Hospital, a medium-size hospital located 30 km south-west of Huddinge. In the area are also located about 40, relatively large, primary healthcare centres which refer patients to HS. The two hospitals, primary healthcare (PHC) providers and the purchaser organisation are the primary stakeholders in the *Star*☆ project.

A.9.2.3 Lombardia

Ospedale Fatebenefratelli e Oftalmico (FBF) is one of oldest hospitals in Milan. It is composed of two distinct areas: the hospital nucleus and the ophthalmic institute. It is extended, with different pavilions, on an area of 27.500 meters. It has 1.600 employees and 300 physicians, with 747 beds.

Azienda U.S.S.L is a Local Healthcare Unit. It has 2.200 employees and an overall turnover of 230 billion Liras (115 million ECU). It manages a population of about 200.000 distributed over 19 municipalities. It includes two hospitals - Busto Arsizio Hospital and Tradate Hospital.

A.9.2.4 Crete

Crete aims towards the development of telematic services improving reliability and effectiveness of the health care system as applied on the island. Crete is a big island with a lot of isolated remote areas which make effective health care delivery very difficult. Patients in remote areas often refer to health care centres and in turn most of them are transferred to the University Hospital of Crete. This results in overloading of patients, thus making appropriate health care delivery very hard. With the application of telematic services unnecessary transfer of patients will be avoided resulting to the improvement care delivery. The main goal of the Paediatric Surgery Clinic of the University Hospital of Crete with *Star*☆ is to provide fast and valuable consulting to GPs in health care centres located in remote areas as well as to enhance the already existing patient record of the clinic with telematic applications and services.

A.9.2.5 Delft

In the Netherlands, *Star*☆ operates in the Delft region connecting almost all GPs in the region, the hospitals, the laboratories, one pharmacy, three medical specialists, home care and health insurer Zorgverzekeraar DSW.

DSW is a public health insurance company, and employs 175 people. Since the beginning of 1992, public health insurance companies are allowed to work nationally, but DSW still concentrates on the region north-west of Rotterdam which has become a leading showcase for healthcare telematics in the Netherlands. People whose annual income is below a certain level are compelled by law to be insured with a public health insurance company for medical treatment necessary for most kinds of illnesses. The insurance package is fixed by law, but each company has its own supplementary fund in which a small additional package is offered.

A.9.2.6 Uusimaa Hospital District

Uusimaa Hospital District represents the Finnish Consortium of Uusimaa Hospital District, Helsinki Health Department and Helsinki University Central Hospital. The satellite work will be performed by Helsinki City Health Department and includes both the primary and secondary care. The City is divided into seven servicing areas of welfare and healthcare. Each area has one hospital, and in total, altogether 32 healthcare stations. There are moreover five specialised hospitals. The aims are to allocate the resources used in the healthcare optimally, and to guarantee:

- fulfilment of the population's requirements on healthcare services;
- care co-ordination of patient groups by avoiding overlaps;
- influence on the time used, costs and the quality of the care process in one unit and between units, which produce seamless care.

Services are provided by primary healthcare units, the secondary care units, the private healthcare units, and the occupational healthcare units. The primary responsibility for care remains in the municipal team, managing primary healthcare on the basis of the principle of the population responsibility.

A.9.2.7 The West Middlesex University Hospital NHS Trust

West Middlesex Hospital provides comprehensive acute care to the London Boroughs of Hounslow and Richmond, serving a local population of approximately 300.000. It currently occupies a 36 acre site, has 450 beds and an annual income of £50m. The Hospital's A&E Department sees 55.000 patients a year, and there are 140.000 outpatient attendances annually. The West Middlesex became an NHS Trust on the 1st April 1993, and employs approximately 2.000 people. The Trust's mission is to provide for its local community a compact, accessible and friendly hospital through which comprehensive acute services are readily available. Included in the strategic direction for the Trust is the need to continue to pay attention to the current and potential markets for its services, and ensure responsiveness to local GPs and patients. This objective accords closely with the *Star*☆ project content. The Trust aims to be responsive to patient, GP, and Health Authority expectations, while ensuring that activity complies with contractual agreements, and seeks to develop the involvement of local GPs and healthcare purchasers in the decision-making process. Already a significant number of healthcare services are provided on a direct-access basis to GPs.

A.9.2.8 Basque Health Service

Osakidetza was created in 1983, becoming the regional health service with full competencies in 1987. Osakidetza has 22.000 employees distributed as follows: physicians 4.629, nurses 10.991, non-medical personnel 5.491 and administration 932. Osakidetza is structured in three public health areas with 14 primary care health districts and a network of 230 hospitals.

A.9.3 Regional partner types

The regional partner types are as follows:

Table D.3: Star regional partner types

Region	Type
North Eastern Health Board	GPs, hospitals and their various services, the regional health authority
Stockholm	Hospitals, primary healthcare providers
Lombardia	Local healthcare unit, hospitals
Crete	GPs in health care centres, paediatric surgery clinics
Delft	Hospitals, laboratories, pharmacy, medical specialists, home care and health insurer
Uusimaa Hospital District	Primary healthcare units, secondary care units, private healthcare units and occupational healthcare units
West Middlesex Hospital	GPs, hospitals
Basque region	Hospitals

A.9.4 Services provided by the project and the technologies used

A.9.4.1 Overview of *Star*☆ Services

The services provided by *Star*☆ comprise:
- Regional services
- Local Services

These are discussed in detail below.

Figure D.19 shows the services that are available now, and the direction being taken by the project to exemplify seamless care:

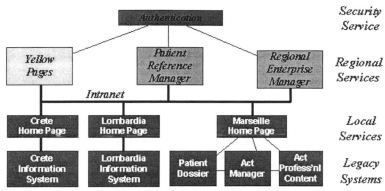

Figure D.19: *Star✩* Services

A.9.4.2 *Star✩* Regional Services

Star✩ Regional Services are the sum of the functionality offered by the Regional Enterprise Manager and Patient Reference Manager.

The scope of the *Star✩* Regional Services is to maintain, at centralised level, a set of references of patient data and healthcare services providers' data, offered to generic clients (users) for enabling exchange and request of information in the healthcare environment.

On top of the services offered by Regional Enterprise Manager and Patient Regional Manager, demonstration applications have been built, allowing the user to perform:

- remote electronic patient record consultation;
- referring a patient;
- booking a health care service for a patient;
- yellow pages, in the sense of organisational and epidemiological information valid outside the inner cycle of care for a patient.

Regional Enterprise Manager

This is devoted to maintaining all the information related to healthcare services providers and single users connected in the network, and can be likened to a "yellow pages" for the healthcare resources in a region. It provides the links for addressing local systems containing the real healthcare data through navigation from the Regional Server. The Regional Enterprise Manager also provides the control and maintenance of all aspects of access, security and privacy of the data and functions through authorisation mechanisms. These may include encryption, passwords, roles or a combination of different data for validation of the request such as smart cards, electronic signature, etc. This has still to be developed according to local needs and final *Star✩* architecture.

Patient Reference Manager

This is devoted to maintaining public demographic information on patients. Detailed (private) data is held on local healthcare providers' systems. In addition it maintains the references of patient contacts enabling a more accurate request and routing of requests. It is clear that authorisation mechanisms in place should be able to filter the "views" of the generic information for the connected clients. The identification of patient by code is left open for each healthcare service providers' systems or modules; it is a function of the Patient Reference Manager to map a patient to the several local patient identifiers that may exist in the network.

Functions provided

The functions offered by the *Star* ☆ Regional Services include at present:
- research functions on patient public data (by authorised users);
- research functions on patient contacts (by authorised users);
- research functions on mixed combination patient-contact (by authorised users);
- research functions on health care service provider, from their location, opening hours, single services providers and their operational details, etc. (public);
- maintenance functions on the data in the two modules (by system administrator and health care service responsible);
- authorisation definition of functions/data accessible for users (by system administrator and health care service responsible);
- routing mechanism for accessing local health care service providers systems from regional server;
- encryption-decryption mechanisms;
- email facilities.

As the presentation (application) is built using HTML pages, any generic internet browser can be connected. All healthcare professional having a modem and a browser for navigation in internet or intranet environment can access the system. The opportunities of access are prioritised for:
- General Practitioners;
- health care professionals working in local units or hospitals or specialised care departments;
- patients, for their own data, plus awareness of healthcare services available in the region.

The benefits deriving from the regional services are:
- a first attempt to provide the core of information necessary for seamless care, overcoming the unsolved problem of direct integration of several incompatible information systems;
- access granted by a generic application (internet web browser) that is widely available at low cost, and has strong commercial support. Web browsers have significant penetration even in the healthcare sector and with confidence already gained;
- the possibility to use services (machines, disk space etc. of third parties) for the definition of regional web, without incurring in great expense;
- scalability and portability of the solution, from a wide environment (internet) to a secure and restricted environment (intranet) without changes in technology;
- global view and promotion of the services offered by providers with increased knowledge;

- routing and address of real location of medical data of the patient, reachable under authorisation, wherever they are distributed;
- more complete aggregated information (as references) of the medical life-cycle of a patient;
- opportunities of inter-organisations collaborations, agreements and contracts for sharing resources and increasing quality of care by overall knowledge of services provided;
- reduction of time (and sometimes impossibility) to retrieve valuable patient information.

A.9.4.3 *Star*☆ Local Services

The *Star*☆ Local Services constitute software modules offering functions (and data management, if necessary) enabling healthcare services providers to publish information from their local systems that is necessary for creating a seamless care network.

Star☆ Local Services work in conjunction with *Star*☆ Regional Services offering information and functions to the users that are addressing them (via the regional servers) for asking or inputting information on patients and care services.

Depending on the openness and information characteristics of the local legacy system of the health care service provider, the *Star*☆ modules could include real physical data.

The purpose of *Star*☆ Local Services is the local publishing for access by external requesters of patient care and service information derived from their registration in legacy systems (if any) and/or enabling a dedicated storage for information for distribution in the network.

The *Star*☆ Local Services include those functions to enable the publication of information references in the regional servers.

The *Star* ☆ Local Services have been developed in three different sites in Europe with the technology available on the site itself, and are all connected and integrated via the Regional Services. Local services are in place in Milan (I), Marseille (F) and Crete (GR).

The *Star*☆ Local Services are developed in the C language (for the functions accessing the data) with presentation in HTML and CGI software for linking the presentation with executable information management programs. These products are independent of the server technical platform and portable to different environments (SUN-Unix servers, Windows NT server) and are functionally independent of the underlying database.

The services are actually based on the (platform independent) web server. Three basic modules have been defined so far:
- Local Enterprise Manager;
- Act Manager;
- Patient Dossier.

Local Enterprise Manager

The Local Enterprise Manager maintains and publishes at a local level all the information regarding the healthcare service provider (organisation) including detailed descriptions of the care services, resources used, protocols applied (medical and administrative) that are considered beneficial for the knowledge of external clients. Moreover, additional local authorisation mechanisms are provided that, in addition to other solutions (e.g. firewalls) can grant security and privacy of the data published in the local system;

Act Manager

The Act Manager maintains registration and tracks the request for services and the services delivered to patients. It also monitors the act life-cycle, from request to performance. In connection with Local Enterprise Manager, it will be able to maintain at a local level all the information necessary for the scheduling of appointments and the booking of care services.

Patient Dossier

The Patient Dossier is a server where the medical information is published that is considered important for seamless care and requested by an authorised third party. It includes patient contacts and diagnostic reports.

The medical data stored are presented accordingly with the limitations of the original legacy system that originated the information. The level of accuracy and completeness of medical data constituting the patient dossier is then variable form site to site, as well as the possibility of developing dedicated applications for exploiting them in the network.

Functions provided

For all the three local services a database is present with the information that can be made available to the network, and is obtained either by interrogating the legacy systems or in an extension of the legacy system itself; in the most favourable case of an open system already structured this way (and therefore compliant with RICHE architectural schema), the modules will just offer the functions to interrogate the local systems. We foresee an intermediate case where there will be a mixed situation between local publishing of information in the *Star*☆ Local Services databases and direct access to legacy systems.

Functions offered by the *Star*☆ Local Services include at present:
- publishing of healthcare service provider organisation and patient demographics and contact reference information, from local to regional servers (by the responsible local system);
- linking contact references information in a value chain for the responsible health care professional of the patient;
- research functions on patient clinical folder, such as ADT abstract, acts executed for the patient and their diagnostic content, presented in different views (by authorised users);
- request for care services by external client and maintenance of act life cycle by performer (by authorised users);

- maintenance functions on the data in the three modules (by system administrator and responsible healthcare service provider);
- API definition for the integration of the *Star*☆ local services with legacy systems;
- authorisation definition of functions/data accessible for users (by local system administrator);
- routing mechanism for accessing local healthcare service providers systems from a regional server;
- encryption-decryption mechanisms;
- emailing facilities.

As the presentation (application) is built using HTML pages, any generic internet browser can be connected.

From this basic set of services, generally valid for all the organisations involved in patient care, dedicated and customised applications exploiting the data managed can be built on the different sites.

These products have been built for the health care services providers that want to participate actively in the health care network, not only accessing external data but also providing data. They will be the key users of the Star☆ telematic services that will build the success of the system by filling it with information.

The client(s)/user(s) typology varies from country to country, dependent on the availability in their premises of electronic information to be shared in the network.
- responsible of hospital/unit information system, managing patient and services data;
- health care professionals working in local units or hospitals or specialised care departments with responsibility (also temporary) for patient medical data;
- General Practitioners having a patient record or scheduling system for their appointments.

Benefits deriving from the local services (excluding applications dedicated to particular functional target):
- sharing information with all the health care participants with clear knowledge benefits;
- receiving requests for services from external sites with the possibility of increasing the market share of the organisation;
- opportunities to expand externally the legacy system in place, adding new functionality and re-organising internal processes;
- empowering inter-organisational relationships;
- developing new opportunities for new services to third parties (i.e. training, epidemiological study, etc.);
- anticipating the health information flow on new wide communication technology as a trend of the market;
- highlighting the position of the organisation in relation to regional/national authorities, offering greater visibility of performance and the improvement of the processes associated with delivering seamless care.

A.9.5 Products resulting from the project

The results of the project can be classified in two groups: software products and consultancy. Below are described the software products, while consultancy will be a potential activity that could be performed in the future due to the know-how acquired in the area and the detailed knowledge of the functionality, IT systems, etc. in the different regions. Moreover, the existence of a regional service over which applications and new services will be implemented, could be a potential area for exploitation for the commercial participants of the project.

The *Star*☆ project software products, as defined and implemented according to the users' requirements, can be split into two main groups:
- *Star*☆ regional services;
- *Star*☆ local services (or *Star*☆ gateway module) that have general applicability for all sites;

plus a third group, called the telematic client applications, which are site-specific and make use of the above services.

The concepts guiding the implementation of these services have been validated by all sites involved in the *Star*☆ project. The portability of the services as well as their scalability have precedence of the final physical architecture for each system. This can range from a small local client-server system, through to a medium sized intranet-based system, up to an internet-wide implementation. The selection of the network infrastructure will be dependent upon the needs of the organisations, their strategies, and the various benefits of seamless care required.

A.9.6 Lessons learnt from the project

The need for networked information systems to support and improve the effectiveness of the delivery of healthcare in Europe, is key part of the Information Society as depicted by the Bangemann Report. In general, healthcare costs continue to rise as a percentage of GDP and there continues to be a significant variation across the European countries despite the intended equal access for European citizens.

Healthcare is an information rich industry. Nonetheless, it continues to invest a significantly lower percentage of expenditure in Information Technology than other comparable sectors. Some of the reasons for this are the changing demographics (ageing population, greater awareness, etc.), improved clinical practices, better quality of care, etc.

The developing informatics market is at a point where it can begin to make a significant impact on the support of healthcare across regions. Many countries have a low-level of healthcare network infrastructure in place and even for those that do, very few are using it for healthcare telematic services. Current healthcare systems are *islands of information* for which *star*☆ can build the bridges. A basic tenet of *star*☆ is to view the information as following the patient's care process, rather than some structured exchange of data between two healthcare agents.

The demonstration of the opportunities exemplified by *star*☆ will enable the healthcare telematics market to significantly grow from the current <2% of healthcare expenditure.

The specific software products that will emerge from the *star*☆ project to contribute to this growth are as follows:

- *star*☆ regional services consisting of:
  - *Regional Enterprise Manager*
  - *Patient Reference Manager*
  - *Security Server*
  - *Public Key Manager*
- *star*☆ local services (or *star*☆ gateway module) that have general applicability for all sites
  - *Act Manager*
  - *Patient Dossier Server*
  - *Local Enterprise Manager*
  - *Booking Server*
- plus a third group, called the *telematic client applications* which are site-specific and make use of the above services

The quantifiable benefits are necessarily complex due to the indirect nature of IT on patient care. Nonetheless, the broad anticipated economic results expected Europe-wide are as follows:

- Gains for the care providers through improved sharing, planning and scheduling of healthcare information and resources resulting in a reduction of cost.
- Gains for the patients through reduced waiting times, length of stay, faster diagnosis, etc.
- Growth for the healthcare informatics industry due to a stimulation of the market resulting from the adoption of open, interoperable, telematic services.
- Growth for the service industry providing value added networked services in healthcare.
- Macro-economic gains due to the improved health of Europe.

Other lessons learned from Star suggest the need for more co-operative ventures between developers. There is much duplication of effort which if streamlined and focussed would yield a much higher level of benefit to citizens who use health services of Europe.